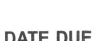 **W9-ALW-813**

DATE DUE

Demco, Inc 38-293

Promoting health in old age

RETHINKING AGEING SERIES

Series editor: Brian Gearing
School of Health and Social Welfare
The Open University

'Open University Press' *Rethinking Ageing* series has yet to put a foot wrong and its latest additions are well up to standard . . . The series is fast becoming an essential part of the canon. If I ever win the lottery, I shall treat myself to the full set in hardback . . .'

Nursing Times

Current and forthcoming titles:
Miriam Bernard: **Promoting health in old age**
Simon Biggs *et al.*: **Elder abuse in perspective**
Ken Blakemore and Margaret Boneham: **Age, race and ethnicity: A comparative approach**
Joanna Bornat (ed.): **Reminiscence reviewed: Perspectives, evaluations and achievements**
Bill Bytheway: **Ageism**
Anthony Chiva and David F. Stears (eds): **Health promotion and older people**
Maureen Crane: **Understanding older homeless people**
Mike Hepworth: **Stories of ageing**
Frances Heywood *et al.*: **Housing and home in later life**
Beverley Hughes: **Older people and community care: Critical theory and practice**
Tom Kitwood: **Dementia reconsidered: The person comes first**
Eric Midwinter: **Pensioned off: Retirement and income examined**
Sheila Peace *et al.*: **Re-evaluating residential care**
Moyra Sidell: **Health in old age: Myth, mystery and management**
Robert Slater: **The psychology of growing old: Looking forward**
John Vincent: **Politics, power and old age**
Alan Walker and Tony Maltby: **Ageing Europe**
Alan Walker and Gerhard Naegele (eds): **The politics of old age in Europe**

Promoting health in old age
Critical issues in self health care

MIRIAM BERNARD

OPEN UNIVERSITY PRESS
Buckingham · Philadelphia

Open University Press
Celtic Court
22 Ballmoor
Buckingham
MK18 1XW

email: enquiries@openup.co.uk
world wide web: http://www.openup.co.uk

and
325 Chestnut Street
Philadelphia, PA 19106, USA

First Published 2000

A catalogue record of this book is available from the British Library

ISBN 0 335 19247 5 (pb)   0 335 19248 3 (hb)

Library of Congress Cataloging-in-Publication Data
Bernard, Miriam.
    Promoting health in old age : critical issues in self health care / Miriam Bernard
        p. cm. – (Rethinking ageing series)
    Includes bibliographical references and index.
    ISBN 0-335-19248-3 (hb.)   ISBN 0-335-19247-5 (pb.)
    1. Aged—Health and hygiene.   2. Self-care. Health.   3. Health promotion.
    I. Title.   II. Series.
    RA564.8.B47   2000
    613'.0438—dc21   99-42447
                                                                                  CIP

Typeset by Type Study, Scarborough
Printed in Great Britain by Biddles Limited, Guildford and Kings Lynn

Contents

Series editor's preface

As the new century begins we are some 15 books into the *Rethinking Ageing* series with several more planned, it seems appropriate to review our original aims in the light of reader responses and the concerns which gave rise to the series. The *Rethinking Ageing* series was planned in the early 1990s, following the rapid growth in ageing populations in Britain and other countries that led to a dramatic increase in academic and professional interest in gerontology. In the 1970s and 80s there had been a steady increase in the publication of British research studies which attempted to define and describe the characteristics and needs of older people. There were also a smaller number of theoretical attempts to reconceptualize what old age means and to explore new ways in which we think about older people. But by the 1990s there was a perception of a widening gap between what was known about ageing from such gerontological research studies, and the limited amount of knowledge and information which was readily available and accessible to the growing number of people with a professional or personal interest in old age. The *Rethinking Ageing* series was conceived as a response to that situation.

The first book to be published in the series was Ken Blakemore and Margaret Boneham's *Age, Race and Ethnicity*. In the series editor's preface we stated that the main aim of the *Rethinking Ageing* series was to fill this knowledge gap with books which would focus on a topic of current concern or interest in ageing (elder abuse, health and illness in later life, dementia etc.). Each book would address two fundamental questions: What is known about this topic? And what are the policy and practice implications of this knowledge? We wanted authors to provide a readable and stimulating review of current knowledge but also to *rethink* their subject area by developing their own ideas in the light of their particular research and experience. We also believed it was essential that the books should be both scholarly and written in clear, non-technical language that would appeal to a broad range of students, academics and professionals with a common interest in ageing and age care.

The books published so far have ranged broadly in subject matter – from ageism to reminiscence to community care to pensions to residential care. The response from individual readers and reviewers has been very positive towards almost all of the titles. The overall success of the series appears to justify the original aims and approach. But how different is the national situation in gerontology ten years on? Compared to even the early 1990s age and ageing are increasingly prominent topics in media and government policy debates. This reflects a greater awareness of the demographic situation – by 2007 there will be more people over pensionable age than there will be children (*The Guardian*, 29 May 1999). However, as a recent article in *Generations Review* noted, despite these developments the number of social gerontology courses are actually (and paradoxically) decreasing (Bernard *et al.*, Vol. 9, No. 3, September 1999). The reasons for this are not straightforward or entirely clear, but they probably reflect the difficulties today's worker-students face in getting sufficient time and funds to attend courses. Alongside this is the pressure on course providers to respond only to the short-term training needs of care staff. Short, problem-focused modules and courses predominate, rather than longer gerontology courses based around an in-depth and truly integrated curriculum that combines the very many different academic disciplines and professional perspectives which contribute to our knowledge and understanding of ageing.

The fact that there appears to be even more interest in ageing and old age than when we started the series persuades us that there is likely to be a continuing need for the serious but accessible topic-based books in gerontology that this series has offered. The uncertainties about the future of gerontology education reinforce this view. However, having already addressed many of the established topic areas in the *Rethinking Ageing* series, we recently felt it was time to extend its subject-matter to include emerging topics or those whose importance has not been widely appreciated. Among the first books to reflect this policy were Maureen Crane's *Understanding Older Homeless People* and John Vincent's *Politics, Power and Old Age*. Miriam Bernard's *Promoting Health in Old Age* combines elements of both the mainstream and the emergent. Whilst focusing on health, a topic of traditional concern to older people, practitioners and policy makers, Bernard's book arises out of an innovative action research project – the Beth Johnson Foundation's Self Health Care in Old Age Programme – which aimed to find new ways of meeting health needs. During the next decade we hope to continue to rethink ageing by revisiting topics already dealt with (via second editions of existing titles) and by finding new titles which can extend the subject matter of the series.

Brian Gearing
School of Health and Social Welfare
The Open University

Preface and acknowledgements

The writing of this book has, as my editor at Open University Press knows only too well, taken a very long time. Its genesis lies in the work I undertook while research officer for the Beth Johnson Foundation, a small voluntary organization which initiates and supports a variety of projects with older people. During the mid-1980s, we became heavily involved in educational work around health issues, establishing the innovative 'Self Health Care in Old Age Project' in 1986. The establishment of this project, together with its associated monitoring and evaluation, forms the core of this book. The project is set in a broader context, through an exploration of the theory, extent and practice of self health care in later life. Bringing together literature from the areas of health education and health promotion, self-help and self-care, and social gerontology, it examines the self health care practices and capacities of older people. It also provides an overview of the main research approaches and developments in this field, drawing on projects from Britain, North America and Israel. In these ways, the book aims to illustrate some of the major issues which confront policy makers and professionals as they strive to understand more fully the part that self health care can play in maintaining the health and well-being of the older population.

This book is, therefore, a synthesis of both practical experience and academic endeavour. It is also the product of a very personal set of circumstances and I have dedicated the book to the memory of my late father and to the continuing energies and insights of my mother. My parents retired and moved to be nearer to us, and my then newly arrived first son, in the autumn after the Self Health Care in Old Age Project was launched. From that time on, they both became involved with aspects of the Foundation's developments: my mother enrolled on one of the early Look After Yourself (LAY) courses and was joined soon afterwards by my father. My father took many of the photographs we used for publicity purposes (some of which are included here) – thus maintaining and using his skills from his career as a professional freelance photographer. Over the years, this involvement was important to them both: initially as a means of making new social contacts and maintaining their own health and well being (my father in particular had suffered with angina for quite some time); and then as an important thread of continuity when my father became very ill some years later. Friends made through the courses stayed in touch during the two years or so that my mother was a full-time carer for my father. Then, when he eventually died just before Christmas 1997, the support was such that my mother found it one of the most natural things to want to return to the group. There, she was welcomed by friends who hugged her and told her very simply that they understood exactly what she had been through, that they shared her sadness and that while life would never again be the same, things would move on.

For me, the intensely personal experience of watching how my parents dealt with the course of my father's developing illness, within the wider context of family and community links, brought home to me exactly the kinds of attitudes and practices we had been trying to achieve through the project. My mother's own account conveys, more vividly than I could ever hope to emulate, the resilience and determination with which they approached this phase in their lives, alongside the difficulties and struggles. With her permission and blessing, I reproduce here what she wrote about this experience:

It began in 1982. Increasingly frequent and severe bouts of indigestion proved to be angina and the start of 15 years of medications, moderations in life style and self help. It seemed under control and we went away, but severe attacks occurred almost daily, aggravated by anxiety and a degree of panic. A doctor at the hotel heard that Cyril was ill, came to us and offered practical advice and reassurance. Back home, we insisted on further investigations and, after this, he was given increased medication and warned that surgery might be indicated. I vividly remember two letters arriving by the same post – one from our doctor striking Cyril off his list, the other for an appointment with a leading cardiac specialist. But, after anxious hours at the hospital we were told there was no question of surgery.

For several years we lived with this – regular medication, low cholesterol diet and extra walking for exercise. Walking uphill became progressively more of a trial, and cold weather aggravated problems so we didn't go out on winter evenings.

In 1986 we retired and moved to be near part of our family. We were fortunate to register with a GP who proved to be exceptional. It was on holiday in 1990 that I realised Cyril, who was by now receiving medication for high cholesterol, had symptoms which could be diabetic. This proved to be correct – he was diagnosed N.I.D. [non-insulin-dependent] and began a regime of more medication and further changes to diet, but arranged to continue treatment through our GP, monitored by home urine tests and regular blood tests at the surgery.

All went well for a while, and we adapted to the common

difficulties of diabetics. I carried the emergency rations and reminded him it was time to eat, but we both suffered when things went awry and he had a hypo and began to sweat and feel faint. Nevertheless, we lived as fully as we could, travelling, going to classes, seeing family and friends.

The diabetes got worse and, in the autumn of 1995, after a full blood picture, there was real bad news – chronic lymphatic leukaemia. Treatment involved weekly visits to the clinic, each with a long wait while blood samples were analysed, and more medication. We asked to be told the truth, so knew that the leukaemia could be controlled but not cured. He still felt ill, and full of aches. Further tests brought more bad news – he had developed haemolytic anaemia and his immune system had turned against him. There was more medication – one drug used for short periods made him feel terrible.

In the spring of 1996 we were allowed a holiday but, soon after we got back and feeling rough after a chest infection, he called in to see our doctor, who at once sent him to hospital. Following assessment he was given a blood transfusion and, after a few days, was allowed home. Within a couple of days his condition deteriorated and he was racked with chest pains. So, it was back into hospital for a 7-unit transfusion and talk of a splenectomy.

This is not the place to tell the story of the Saturday night panic when the blood ran out and the remaining units were 'lost', but it was a time of the utmost emotional and physical stress. He came out of hospital in a very poor state – purple with bruising all over his body and so weak that it was only with the greatest determination that he got upstairs with my help. Although we moved a bed into the lounge for daytime rest, he insisted on getting upstairs to bed, and to shave and dress every day. But then he got so weak that this was impossible.

He was determined not to go back into hospital for anything, and not to have a splenectomy which carried high risks for him. With our doctor's cooperation, we all agreed he would be looked after at home. Again, we asked for the truth, and learned that he might have six months left. At this point, and in view of his state – depressed in every sense – he was prescribed morphine and agreed to visits from a nurse specialist in palliative care from the local hospice.

Unexpectedly, he began to improve and to fight back. By the end of the six months he was able to travel again, and we managed to go away for a weekend. There were many problems, many adjustments, some conflicts. It was difficult at times to support him in what he wanted to do, but this was essential for his confidence and integrity. We tried to make the best of every day, and to do whatever we could, whenever he felt well enough. The support of our family, friends, doctor and nurse were essential in sustaining the remission which gave us an extra, worthwhile year (but which had its own crisis when he developed pneumonia – also successfully treated at home).

Unbelievably, in the autumn of 1997, we managed to go to Spain for a week. His courage and determination carried him through but when we got back, he was an exhausted, frail, sick man and we knew it wouldn't be long. Eventually it all became too much for him to manage. A week before Christmas, he decided to go into the hospice for assessment, but died in his sleep five days later.

It is my hope that readers of this book will learn something of what it is actually like to engage in the kinds of self health care practices vividly expressed in my mother's account, but also through the experiences recalled by many of the older participants and volunteers who will be encountered in the following pages.

In writing this book, I have been fortunate to come into contact with a wide range of people to whom I owe a considerable debt of gratitude. First, I must acknowledge the many many older people with whom I have worked since I first stumbled quite by accident into gerontology in 1982. Their enthusiasm and optimism for what we were doing gave me the courage to continue down this road when sceptics questioned my sanity about 'what a young woman like you is doing in a field like this'! Second, my special thanks go to Dr Frank Glendenning who, as chair of the Beth Johnson Foundation, took the ultimate leap of faith in appointing a callow Geography and English graduate to the vacant post of research officer. As mentor, colleague and friend Frank has been a constant and much valued presence in my life. To my colleagues during the time I was at the Foundation: particularly Arthur Creber (Director) and Vera Ivers (Principal Officer – Development), I am forever indebted. Their belief and trust in me was undoubtedly key to my own development as a gerontologist, and I hope they feel that I have done justice to the creative years we were all together.

Over the years, I have also met and talked to colleagues around the world who are engaged in similar research and developments to those I discuss in this book. A number of them have commented on parts of this text, sent me information and words of encouragement. In this context, I must first acknowledge my good friend and colleague Kathy Meade, but also Meredith Minkler from the University of California, Sandra Cusack from Simon Fraser University in Vancouver, Beryl Petty from Century House, Ilana Mizrahi and her research colleagues from the Brookdale Institute in Jerusalem, and Yosefa Ben-Moshe from Eshel: the Association for Planning and Development for the Elderly in Israel. Since taking up my post at Keele University in 1988, past and present colleagues have provided support and a stimulating intellectual environment in which to develop these, and other, ideas to the full. Long may we continue to do so! My appreciation also goes, as ever, to the many students on our gerontology courses. For a decade now, it has been my privilege to present some of the ideas and views debated here to these most discerning and reflective of 'consumers', at both undergraduate and postgraduate levels.

Thanks go too to other colleagues, but particularly to Gilly Crosby at the Centre for Policy on Ageing, who has always willingly tracked down elusive references for me; to Professor John Benington, who, as the external evaluator on the project, urged us to have the courage of our convictions and to pursue the action research route to the full; and to Sue Allingham, for her help with the final stages of this manuscript and especially for her continuing, and daily, support.

Last but by no means least, it is customary on these occasions to record the disruptions to family life and the fortitude of close family. For me, this period of my life has truly been a family affair – my eldest son Jacob was born in the summer the project came into being, and I have pictures of him at just over a month old at the official opening of the Senior Health Shop. My youngest son Ben was born four years later just as the initial European funding for the project was coming to an end. My parents – Cyril and Margaret – were early participants in the project, and my partner Steve has, in very recent months, taken on the task of monitoring and evaluating the Foundation's newest developments in intergenerational work. For us all, self health care has been a constant reality as well as a research-based endeavour!

Finally, my appreciation goes to the people at Open University Press who have held faith with me in the belief that this book would eventually see the light of day. Brian Gearing offered constructive criticism in the latter stages and, to Jacinta Evans, Editorial Director, and Joan Malherbe, Senior Editorial Assistant, your persistent cajoling and encouragement has at long last, I hope, been vindicated.

1

The challenge of an ageing population

Introduction

At the start of the new millennium, the ageing of the UK population is one of the most important challenges to be faced. While the prolongation of a healthy life and the prevention of disabling diseases are undisputedly desirable goals, the recognition that there is scope for older people themselves to improve their health has been a long time in coming. However, during the 1980s and 1990s, there was growing interest and mounting activity in Britain around health issues, with older people being a key group in these developments (Bernard and Phillipson 1991).

The growth of health promotion generally, and the development of the Beth Johnson Foundation's Self Health Care in Old Age Project in particular, form the focus of this book. My argument is that although self health care is crucial to the maintenance of health and well-being, and has long been the most extensive and basic form of health care, its potential has been seriously neglected when considering later life. The task of this opening chapter, therefore, is to set the scene by examining the historical context which led to increasing interest in the health of older people in the latter part of the twentieth century. It first highlights the complexity of this issue and looks at how we, as a society, view older people. It then goes on to examine socio-demographic trends and the implications of these for the health status of older people. This is followed by a consideration of the resources and structures within which health is delivered, looking at the development of the National Health Service (NHS) and of primary health care in particular. The chapter concludes by emphasizing a number of key issues which underpin this whole area of concern.

More detailed discussions of the emergence and role of health promotion with older people will be found in Chapter 2 before moving on to look at the research and practice of self health care in Chapters 3 and 4. Together, these first four chapters provide the broad historical, conceptual and policy context against which to set our examination of the Self Health Care in Old Age Project. Described by Sidell (1995: 128) as 'one of the best examples' aimed at improving the health and well-being of older people, the second half of the book illustrates how the research, ideas and developments discussed in preceding chapters can be made to work in practice, and what impact such a development has on the health and lifestyles of participants, volunteers and staff. The final chapter draws together the empirical findings with the earlier analyses, in order to highlight the relevance of such developments to current policy and practice.

Thinking about health and old age

The maintenance of health and well-being in later as in earlier life is a very complex, not to say contentious issue. The reasons for this are many and varied and have to do with what Sidell (1995) has eloquently described as the myths and mysteries surrounding the relationship of health to old age. The myths she identifies include:

- the notion of 'the elderly' as a homogeneous group – who share common characteristics and who can therefore be regarded as if they were all the same;
- the 'medical myth' – which perpetuates the idea that growing older is synonymous with disease and ill health;
- the mortality–morbidity debate – which claims that death is increasingly concentrated in the later years, and that people will remain fitter and healthier for longer before they die;
- the emergence of the 'super oldie' – a seemingly positive image but one which, in reality, may be just as oppressive as the medical myth.

To these she adds a number of mysteries:

- why it is that women live longer, but tend to suffer with more chronic and disabling diseases than men;
- where the responsibility for health lies: with the individual, the medical profession or the welfare state;
- why older people are an anomalous group in that they subjectively rate their health as good in the face of seemingly contradictory objective evidence;
- what it is we mean by health.

These link closely with two further issues which Henwood (1990) has argued work against older people maintaining good health. These are:

- the assumptions which we have about the quality of health which can be expected in old age;
- discrimination against older people in the provision of health care.

Together, these issues are fundamental to the discussions about health in general and self health care in particular. It is hoped that readers of this book do not have to be convinced that old age is not itself a disease, nor are many of the associated conditions either inevitable or universal. Yet, this presents us with crucial dilemmas when we look at the relationship between health and older people, and the societal context of that relationship. How in fact do we tread those fine lines between promoting and encouraging individual responsibility for health but without letting it tip over into victim blaming; between state provision and individual or informal health care; between the health needs of older people and those of other groups; between an emphasis on treating sickness or on promoting health; and between getting the conditions and problems which older people suffer from taken seriously, but without it contributing adversely to further negative stereotyping? These are undoubtedly difficult issues but one way forward is to begin by looking at what we know about population ageing, and about older people and their health.

Population ageing

Britain, together with many other western industrialized nations, is in the vanguard of the ageing process. During the twentieth century, both the numbers and the proportions of people we now term 'elderly' increased dramatically. It is these increases that have given rise to the term 'an ageing population'. Historically, Britain has never before had such an elderly population (Laslett 1996), and this situation will become even more marked in the new millennium.

Population ageing has occurred with great rapidity throughout the twentieth century. The major factor accounting for this has been declining fertility: the UK population is not ageing primarily because we are living longer (although we are) but because, crudely, we are producing fewer babies per woman. Coupled with this, we have also experienced declining mortality rates (notably infant and child mortality), alongside an increase in the expectation of life. Life expectation has risen steadily for both males and females, although the increases have been greatest for women. In 1901, life expectation at birth was 48 years for men and 52 years for women, figures which had not in fact shown any improvement since medieval times. In 1995, women had gained 27 years and could expect to live until about the age of 79, while men had gained 25 years and could expect to live until about the age of 73 (Office for National Statistics (ONS) 1996). Life expectation is still rising, but the differential gap between men and women is predicted to close slightly in the future.

While the ageing of the population is clearly evident at a societal level, we also have to be aware of the fact that the older segment of our population is itself ageing. This has been most marked during the 1970s, 1980s and 1990s. However, although the total pensionable population is projected to grow fairly slowly in the short term, longer term forecasts about the projected increases in the numbers of people aged 75 and over, and 85 and over, suggest that the former will double in size by the middle of the twenty-first century, and the latter will triple (Office of Population Censuses and Surveys (OPCS) 1997). Indeed, the older the age group one considers, the greater the forecast percentage increases are. The growth of centenarians is perhaps the clearest indication of this trend, with their ranks being expected to swell from a total of 8000 people in 1999 (7000 women and 1000 men), to 34,000 (28,000 women and 6000 men) by 2031 (OPCS 1997).

This ageing of the population obviously has implications for health, and indeed for other social and welfare practices and policies. Yet, although Britain's population will continue to age in the twenty-first century, it is important to view this continuing demographic challenge in tandem with other changes in the social, economic and political circumstances society is undergoing and which impact on older, as on younger, people (Wells and Freer 1988; Bernard and Phillips 1998). What then, at the start of the twenty-first century, does Britain's ageing population look like, and what changes might we realistically expect?

Older people in Britain

At the start of the twentieth century, Britain had some 2 million people of pensionable age, who accounted for about 5 per cent of the total population. By 1951, the proportion of the population who were 'elderly' had risen to 14 per cent and by 1995 it was over 18 per cent – in other words, almost one in five people are over pensionable age (ONS 1996). The 10.5 million elderly people alive in Britain means that the twentieth century witnessed a fivefold increase in terms of absolute numbers. A related point to consider is that later life is, and will remain in simple numerical terms, primarily an experience of women. Two-thirds of those of pensionable age are women and one-third are men, with ageing becoming a progressively gendered experience such that at age 75 and over, women outnumber men by two to one; at age 85 and over by four to one; and, at the age of 100, by seven to one (OPCS 1997). This 'feminization of later life', as it has been termed (Arber and Ginn 1991), is further reflected in other related socio-demographic characteristics such as marital status and living arrangements.

There are increasing numbers of widows and widowers in old age, while the rise of solo living has become ever more prominent (Evandrou 1998). Currently, nearly half of older women are either single or married, with the other 50 per cent being widowed. This contrasts with only 17 per cent of men who are widowers (ONS 1996). The experience of widowhood also increases with increasing age and, by the time women reach 85 years of age, over three-quarters of them will be in this situation. Moreover, half of women over the age of 65 live alone compared with only 20 per cent of men. As a consequence of other changes, notably predicted increases in separation and divorce, this tendency to live alone in old age is predicted to go on increasing for both men and women (Falkingham 1997). We also know that lone elderly people are considerably under-represented among owner occupiers and over-represented in the rented sector, and that they tend to reside in the worst housing conditions with significant minorities still lacking amenities such as a bath, an inside toilet or central heating (Peace and Johnson 1998).

A further important dimension of socio-demographic change is the growth in numbers of black and minority ethnic elders. Currently, the percentages are relatively small: typically only 2 or 3 per cent. However, census comparisons and demographic trends suggest that although minority ethnic groups have what is termed a 'young age profile', the coming decades will witness a marked growth, particularly in the numbers of older people of Asian and African Caribbean origin, as those now in middle age get older. Given associated influences such as the geographical distribution of these groups, changing family structures and the myths and assumptions surrounding family care giving, it is evident that meeting the particular health and social care needs of minority ethnic elders and planning appropriate and accessible services, will become a matter of increasing importance. Indeed, the numbers can now no longer be dismissed as being too small to cause concern in respect of policy and practice (Atkin 1998).

In sum, older people now find themselves in a very diverse set of circumstances, in contrast to the myth of homogeneity highlighted earlier. Alterations to the structure of our population have been accompanied by profound changes in the size and composition of the family, as the effects of lowered fertility and increasing divorce begin to make their impact felt on the older generations (Bernard and Phillips 1998). Moreover, the dramatic changes which have been wrought to the age structure of Britain's population over the twentieth century are not temporary – they are not some statistical aberration – they are permanent gains for humankind, and we should regard it as a matter for celebration that more and more people are surviving into later life (Jefferys 1988). The key features of these changes include the rapidity with which our population has aged; the ageing of the elderly population itself; the feminization of later life; the changes in marital status and living arrangements; and the growing numbers of black and minority ethnic elders. These features raise innumerable challenges for us in relation to health, and it is to this that we now turn.

Older people and health

The medical myth referred to earlier has perpetuated the idea that growing older is inevitably linked with disease and disability and has resulted in the bleak but popular and all powerful image of health in old age, described by Scrutton (1992) as:

> One associated with an increase in pain, discomfort, illness, disease and dependence; loss of energy and personal drive; significantly greater need for rest; long and increasing periods of sickness; permanent experience of pain and discomfort; increasing immobility; the gradual loss of personal control and responsibility; the onset of incontinence, with resulting loss of dignity and self-respect; increasing confusion; and, ultimately, the most feared condition of all, senility.
>
> (Scrutton 1992: 10)

Such is the dominance of this view that it has, in turn, contributed to much research on the health of older people being not about health at all, but about the prevalence of ill health and about specific medical conditions (Victor

1991). It is not, however, the purpose of this discussion to detail the conditions from which older people suffer; readers with particular interests in this perspective can find explanations in numerous other texts (see for example Bennett and Ebrahim 1995). Rather, this discussion begins from the premise that articulating what it is that older people mean when they talk about being healthy is important both for the kinds of health promotion activities which form the core of this book, and for formulating policy objectives which can be translated into successful practice.

Thus, we begin by looking first at how health is conceptualized and understood for, as Sidell (1995: xix) argues: '"Ways of seeing" affect "ways of knowing" and health is a much contested concept.' We then go on to explore some of the paradoxes and dilemmas which exist around health and older people. In particular, we look at acute and chronic health problems and at functional disability in an attempt to illuminate why it is, in Nathanson's (1977) words, 'women get sick, but men die'. In addition, this will also help shed light on how and why older people's subjective ratings of their health status seem to be at odds with more objective evidence. This part of the discussion will conclude with a look at the future in terms of the mortality–morbidity debate.

Being healthy

For older as for younger people, health is crucial to the maintenance of well-being. However, in much the same way as our views of ageing and old age are socially and economically structured, so too are our ideas about what it is to be healthy (Sidell 1993). It is a difficult concept to pin down and many commentators have pointed to the variations and differing implications which arise, according to whether we look at lay perspectives (that is bottom-up, from ordinary people) as opposed to professional perspectives (that is top-down and official) (Victor 1991; Jones 1994; Sidell 1995; Hardey 1998). Ever since the World Health Organization (WHO 1948) defined health as 'not merely the absence of disease and infirmity but complete physical, mental and social well-being', the literature has become replete with debates about whether health should be defined negatively as the absence of disease, or more positively and holistically. In reality, as Hardey (1998) notes, both dimensions find empirical support from studies which have looked at lay ideas about health. However, the disease oriented perspective is strongly sanctioned in Britain by the tendency to rely on mortality and morbidity statistics as indicators of health, and to build national strategies and policies around targets designed to reduce ill health and disease under the guise of improving the health of the nation. Concentrating on death and disease in this way, while it may be used as a proxy for health, is very negative in that it tells us nothing about how people subjectively experience being healthy, how they cope with illness or disease, or how these terms may contrast or coexist with one another.

Studies in the UK and elsewhere have shown that beliefs and attitudes about health are 'complex, inconsistent, dynamic and fragmentary' (Hardey 1998: 29). They are based on people's values and expectations, and linked with social and cultural situations. Since Herzlich (1973) first explored how people define health and illness in the early 1970s, there has been a gradual accumulation of research on these topics using a variety of both quantitative and qualitative methodologies (R.G.A. Williams 1981, 1983; Pill and Stott 1982, 1985; Blaxter 1983, 1990; Cornwell 1984; Calnan 1987; Wenger 1988; Stainton-Rogers 1991; Backett and Davison 1992). Generally speaking, a synthesis of this literature seems to suggest that the lay population identify three broad dimensions to health: the absence of disease/not being ill; being functionally fit/coping with daily activities; and as a state of positive fitness (Victor 1991: 95). Variations and interactions are observable too with regard to dimensions such as class, gender, race, socio-economic status, living environments, cultural and religious beliefs, and age. A further complication, as Jones (1997b: 24) observes, is not only that different groups of people define health in different or similar ways, but also that 'the same person may use several distinctive explanations or stories to make up a complete account'. This was certainly the case in Sidell's (1991: 28) qualitative interviews with older women when, typically, 'they would express sometimes conflicting beliefs and attitudes at different points in the conversation'.

Notwithstanding the above complexities, we do find that there is a greater tendency for older people to view health in functional terms, emphasizing the importance of resilience and of being able to cope, rather than fitness (Blaxter and Paterson 1982; R.G.A. Williams 1983, 1990; Blaxter 1990; Jones 1997b). In addition, the Health and Lifestyle Survey (Blaxter 1990) reveals that when asked what it felt like when they were healthy, well over half of the older men and women responded by saying that health was about 'feeling good'. This emotional/psychological aspect was articulated with phrases such as 'being happy', 'being unstressed' and 'being able to cope' (Victor 1991: 97). These findings echo Rory Williams's (1983, 1990) work with older Aberdonians, Cornwell's (1984) work in the East End of London, and Sidell's (1991) study on gender differences in health at older ages. However, the research also begs other questions, such as to what extent these conceptions are framed by Henwood's (1990) argument about the assumptions that we have about the quality of health which can be expected in old age, and whether this will change in the future as younger cohorts have greater opportunities to be involved in health education and promotion. Succeeding chapters will attempt to address these issues further, but we turn now to look at the state of health of people who are old today, examining how healthy they think they are from both subjective and objective viewpoints.

How healthy are older people?

We have already noted the anomaly inherent in using mortality statistics to examine the health of older people. Yet, trends in late life mortality are an important part of the overall picture. In Britain, mortality rates for middle aged and older women have fallen continuously since the start of the twentieth century (Grimley Evans *et al.*1992). For men, this decline was marred from the 1930s to the 1970s due to increases from coronary heart disease and smoking-related diseases (Grimley Evans *et al.* 1992; Grimley Evans 1998). More recently though, improvements in male mortality have been greater than for women, with trends in smoking being the most strongly implicated reason (Sidell 1995). Despite this, the major causes of death are the same for both older men and women, with cardiovascular and respiratory diseases being the leading causes, alongside cancers and cerebrovascular disorders. The discernible gender differences are related more to the sites of cancers, and to the pace of death (Verbrugge 1989). Other authors have further shown how class, race and ethnicity impact on mortality rates, with the inequalities and differentials that are discernible earlier in life persisting well into old age (Estes *et al.* 1984; Marmot *et al.* 1984; Fox *et al.* 1985; Townsend and Davidson 1986; Whitehead 1987; Townsend *et al.* 1988; Raleigh *et al.* 1996; Balarajan and Raleigh 1997). It is also the case that the risk factors for many of the leading causes of death are now so well known that the argument for taking a positive, preventive approach is clear, and would provide a much needed corrective to the notion that where older people's health is concerned, they are simply a continuing financial drain and burden on the rest of society (Iliffe *et al.* 1998; Johnson 1998; Warnes 1998).

While age specific mortality rates have declined and life expectation has increased, the most important area still to consider concerns the extent of morbidity, illness and disability among the older population. There are various sources we can draw on here but much of our information comes from the General Household Survey which, since 1980, has included special sections on people aged 65 and over (Iliffe *et al.* 1998). Included among the questions, the General Household Survey asks respondents if they have any *longstanding* illness, disability or infirmity. Those who say yes are then asked if it limits their activities in any way (subsequently called a longstanding limiting illness). What we find is that three-fifths or more of both older men and women have such an illness, and that the prevalence increases with advancing age (OPCS 1995). More women than men are affected, although not everyone with a longstanding illness goes on to say that it restricts their activity. Following our earlier discussions about what health is, this suggests that it may be possible to define oneself as healthy even in the presence of illness or disability.

In terms of *functional disability* and chronic health problems, the General Household Survey also provides information about whether or not people can perform various activities of daily living such as those associated with mobility (for example walking outside or getting up and down stairs), self-care tasks (such as bathing and washing) and domestic tasks (for instance shopping and cooking). This reveals that older women have higher levels of physical incapacity than men. For example, Arber and Ginn (1991) report that among people aged 75 and over, twice as many women as men are housebound (22 per cent compared with 11 per cent). More recent data confirm this and show that nearly half of women over the age of 85 are unable to perform one or more activities such as going out and walking down the road on their own, getting up and down stairs, or getting around the house (OPCS 1996).

Older women are also less able than older men to carry out personal self-care tasks (Ginn and Arber 1998), although it must be remembered that we are talking here about minorities of older people. Indeed, 1991 data show that fully four-fifths of men and women over the age of 85 are still able to feed themselves, get in and out of bed, bathe themselves and get to the toilet without help, and that these figures are in fact a substantive improvement over the previous decade (Grundy 1996). In relation to domestic activities, Arber and Ginn (1991) also make the important observation that cultural assumptions about gender role behaviour are likely to influence findings because men are much more likely than women to receive help with these tasks in old age. A further issue is that these prevalence rates may well be underestimates because the General Household Survey data do not take into account older people living in institutional settings who, almost by definition, will have higher rates of disability (Grundy 1998).

Findings about the prevalence of longstanding illness, chronic health problems and disability also lead us to consider just what kinds of disorders result in these observable gender and age differences. Iliffe and his colleagues (1998: 4) list the major causes of disability as cardiovascular diseases (including cerebrovascular disorders), loss of vision and hearing, osteoarthritis, osteoporosis, urinary incontinence, depression and dementia: this list is confirmed by other national data sets and studies such as the Health and Lifestyles Survey (Cox *et al.* 1987), the Carnegie Inquiry into the Third Age (Grimley Evans *et al.* 1992) and the Health Survey for England (OPCS 1995). Some marked gender differences occur, particularly in relation to the already observed high prevalence of heart and circulatory disorders among men, and the difficulties which women experience with musculoskeletal problems including arthritis and painful joints (Grundy 1998).

Such gender and age differences are also observable in self-reports of the prevalence of acute health problems (Victor 1991). The Health and Lifestyle Survey (Cox *et al.* 1987), for example, shows not only that women report considerably more symptoms, but also that the widest gender differences occur in relation to pains in the joints, headaches, and trouble with eyes and feet. The latter also show marked increases with advancing age. As well as these physical symptoms, the Health and Lifestyle Survey adapted the General Health Questionnaire (Goldberg 1972) to develop what they called a malaise index. Again, we find marked gender differences with older women reporting more symptoms than men for all categories – difficulty in sleeping, and worrying being particularly notable. On the whole then, we can conclude that older women, much more so than older men, tend to accumulate highly symptomatic, but non-lethal, diseases and conditions (Sidell 1995).

Race and ethnicity further confound this picture. Although there is some evidence for higher rates of mortality for certain conditions and diseases (Balarajan 1995; Raleigh *et al.* 1996; Balarajan and Raleigh 1997) and the reporting of poorer health in comparison with the white population (Rudat 1994; Silveira and Ebrahim 1995), there are a number of observations and caveats to be made here. First, the gender balance among minority ethnic groups is not necessarily the same as among white elders. For example, the ratio for African Caribbeans is similar, but there are more older men than women in South Asian populations (Atkin 1998). Second, we lack a comprehensive national picture of the extent, nature or experience of chronic illness or disability among minority ethnic groups, with the result that the information we do have has to be pieced together from small-scale and local surveys (Blakemore and Boneham 1993; Douglas 1997; Atkin 1998). Third, while there is a growth of interest in specific conditions and in studies examining the incidence of disability (Royal Association for Disability and Rehabilitation (RADAR) 1984; Greater London Association for Disabled People (GLAD) 1987; NHS Centre for Reviews and Dissemination 1996), work on issues such as mental infirmity is notable by its absence (Silveira and Ebrahim 1995). Given the present dearth of information, it is vitally important not to regard black and minority ethnic elders as a homogeneous group: there are differences among different ethnic groups in, for example, rates of limiting longstanding illness (Charlton *et al.* 1994; Evandrou 1996; Nazroo 1997), as well as similarities with white elders. These cautions apply too as we go on to consider additional aspects, such as older people's subjective perceptions of their health status, the use that older people make of existing services, and the responses they receive from health and social care professionals.

Perceptions of health

From the surveys discussed above, we also know something about how older people assess health status: both their own, and in comparison with other people. We saw earlier that three-fifths of older men and women suffer from some form of chronic longstanding illness or disability, and that substantive proportions of older women have high levels of functional incapacity, mental malaise and acute health problems. Yet, when assessing their health status, two-fifths of older people rate their health as 'good', although women are somewhat less optimistic about this than men (Midwinter 1991; Victor 1991; Sidell 1995). Moreover, with increasing age, both sexes tend to switch their health rating from good to fairly good.

Although a great deal of self-assessed health status tallies with objective measures, there is an anomaly here in that considerable minorities of older people persist in defining themselves as in good health in the face of contradictory evidence. We find this in both survey data, and in qualitative studies (Wenger 1988; Midwinter 1991; Sidell 1991). Explanations seem to relate to the tendency for older people to see themselves as in better health than their peers and as well enough to carry out their necessary activities (Cockerham *et al.* 1983); to want not to define themselves as ill and to keep going (R.G.A. Williams 1981, 1983); and to minimize health problems and not admit publicly to being unwell (Cornwell 1984; Wenger 1988). Whatever explanation we might favour, or data we choose to draw on, this reaffirms just how complex a subject the health of older people is, and how important it is not to fall into the trap of classifying them as ill, diseased or healthy without a proper grasp of how people conceptualize, understand and experience these terms.

A healthy later life?

Alongside the need to think further about the ways in which we view health, illness and disease, the literature of recent years has also emphasized the importance of devising ways which measure what has been variously termed active life expectancy (ALE), healthy active life expectancy (HALE) or expectation of life without disability (ELWD) (Grimley Evans *et al.* 1992; Grimley Evans 1993, 1998; Bone *et al.* 1995). The search for such measures has been prompted by the debate which has been going on since the 1960s concerning whether or not increasing life expectancy will be accompanied by better, or worse, health. This mortality–morbidity debate basically comprises two opposing views: one predicts a continued concentration of death in the later years (the rectangularization of mortality) with a concomitant decrease in the incidence of disabilities among the older population and their occurrence only during the last few years of life (the compression of morbidity); the other predicts substantial increases of very old people, many of whom will be suffering from chronic conditions and will simply be kept alive for longer (Bury 1988; Rogers *et al.* 1990).

Fries and Crapo take the optimistic view and argue from the basis that the human lifespan is fixed at around 85 years of age (Fries 1980; Fries and Crapo 1981). Their initial proposals were based on the contention that as a species, we are reaching the upper limit of our survival potential and that mortality improvements have led to increasingly rectangular survival curves. In other words, premature death has been reduced and more and more people are surviving into their eighties with the body finally wearing out at the end of the natural lifespan rather than succumbing to disease. Fries went on to argue that while western society may have been successful in controlling premature death, the challenge we now face concerns how to deal with longer periods dominated by chronic disease.

Using the case of two brothers – one of whom is a heavy smoker, while the other is a light smoker – he also suggested that it was possible, through preventive health practices and associated interventions, to postpone the onset of many chronic diseases. At the beginning of the twentieth century, the heavy smoker would have been quite likely, at around the age of 30, to have contracted pneumonia and died prematurely after an illness lasting perhaps for only three days. Nowadays Fries argues that, with penicillin, this man would survive pneumonia but at about the age of 40 he might develop a cough, wheezing and shortness of breath. If he continues to smoke he will be increasingly short of breath for the rest of his life. In his fifties he may have a heart attack. Again, prior to modern high-tech medicine it is likely that he would have died at this point. This is now controllable, although he might then go on to have a stroke a few years later involving considerable rehabilitation. Throughout, he remains short of breath and, finally, he develops lung cancer and dies in his seventies.

In contrast, the lighter smoking brother does not develop emphysema until much later in life – perhaps not until he is about 70. The heart attack is postponed as is the stroke, but he dies at the limit of his lifespan and does not succumb to the lung cancer at all.

What Fries is arguing is that *if* the onset of such chronic diseases can be postponed by preventive health care measures, by better use of health services, and by increasing personal responsibility for one's own health, then what is known as the 'compression of morbidity' will occur alongside the 'rectangularisation of mortality' (Bury 1988). Instead of lingering with chronic illness for many years like the first brother, individuals will be more vigorous for longer. From this basis, Fries is very optimistic about the future state of health of the older population. Indeed, since he first articulated his propositions in 1980 he has, with research colleagues at the Stanford Arthritis Center in California, undertaken numerous studies to examine and test this hypothesis. Since the mid-1980s in particular, they have been concerned with exploring the health benefits of long distance running (Lane *et al.* 1986, 1987, 1990; Fries *et al.* 1994). Alongside this, they have written about the relationship of age and gender to morbidity (Leigh and Fries 1994), while Fries himself has continued to argue that the compression of morbidity paradigm is an important policy strategy in the pursuit of cutting health care costs and extending disability-free life expectancy (Fries 1990, 1993, 1996).

Not surprisingly, Fries's early formulation was challenged, with a number of authors contesting that there was no empirical evidence to support his assumption that the human lifespan is fixed (Bytheway 1982; Manton 1982; Schneider and Brody 1983). Moreover, with regard to the compression of morbidity issue, Fries's opponents were, and still are, sceptical of his claims about whether or not the onset of chronic illness can be postponed (Bury 1988). Alternative interpretations even go so far as to anticipate that older populations will become less healthy, with alarming projections of the numbers who will be chronically ill and require long-term care, alongside increasing numbers who will be widowed, disabled and socially isolated – what has been graphically termed 'the increasing misery' scenario (Verbrugge 1984; Manton 1986; Olshansky *et al.* 1991). Some commentators further argue that the compression of morbidity paradigm, while it may fit with the experiences of older men, is inappropriate with regard to the situations of older women (Verbrugge 1984, 1989; Lewis 1985; Sidell 1991). Criticisms have also been levelled at the conception of dependency and disability as irreversible, with a focus on delaying onset diverting attention from the possibility that recovery may also extend disability-free life expectancy (Rogers *et al.* 1990).

The debate continues to flourish, partly because current evidence is unable to conclusively prove or disprove that morbidity compression is possible and partly because there is some basis for both views (Bone *et al.* 1995). In fact, it is also suggested that it is quite possible that both phenomena will be taking place simultaneously: that there may be an increasing proportion of individuals in quite good health up to the point of death and an increasing proportion with prolonged severe functional limitations. The proportion suffering from only a moderate degree of infirmity is therefore likely to decline. Part of the problem lies with the nature of the data we have because many of the studies of longevity and health are cross-sectional and often lead to the conclusion that increases in length of life are not matched by increases in healthy life (Bebbington 1988; Crimmins *et al.* 1989). Optimistically though, some longitudinal US data are beginning to show that average lifespan is increasing and that disability in later life is falling (Manton and Stallard 1994; Manton *et al.* 1997). Although this may not be happening as fast as Fries and his colleagues predicted, it has led to the observation that 'modest optimism seems to have better justification than panic' (Tallis 1998: vii).

However uncertain or debatable the future, the evidence we have to date surely points, as Bond and Coleman (1993: 338) argue, towards a need to turn our attention seriously 'to identifying ways of preventing ill health and maintaining health in elderly people'. Before doing this in Chapter 2, one further piece of the jigsaw needs to be added to our current exploration of the health status of older people. This concerns whether the diversity and complexity we have been discussing are also reflected in the use made of health services by older men and women, and how professionals working in the system respond to their health needs. It is to these issues that we now turn.

Health care services

Quite clearly, issues about the extent of disability and dependency among older people are at the heart of policy debates about how best to meet their health needs. Yet here again we are having to tread one of those very fine lines because it is important to remind ourselves that although only minorities of older people (albeit substantial minorities) suffer with chronic and disabling conditions and acute illnesses, they record the highest per capita expenditure in simple age-related terms, and are the major recipients of health and social welfare services (Robinson and Judge 1987; Victor 1991; Office of Health Economics (OHE) 1995; Dalley 1998). This is despite the fact that when we look at health expenditure by type of care provided, specialist services for older people currently come well down the list in terms of resourcing, along with services for mentally ill, mentally handicapped and physically disabled people (Victor 1991).

Moreover, continuing policy shifts, including the introduction of internal markets and the series of reorganizations leading up to the most recent changes in the wake of the National Health Service and Community Care Act 1990, mean that older people's experiences of the NHS have been variable to say the least (Dalley 1998). It has also led some critics to argue that the NHS has treated older people particularly badly (Webster 1991) with attempts to reduce expenditure and cut long-stay beds, impacting most strongly on older age groups (Victor 1991). Set against this, however, it is important to recognize that the creation of the NHS in 1948 also enabled older people to deal with chronic illness in ways which had been impossible before the Second World War, and thus to live healthier lives than they had previously (Hardey 1998). Undoubtedly too, older people have also benefited from the achievements of medical science and its technological advances, from developments in the treatment of particular diseases and conditions, and from the strides made in palliative care (Dalley 1998). Yet even at the end of the twentieth century, there is still considerable concern about the way older people are dis-advantaged, discriminated against and responded to, in terms of health care practice and policy (Scrutton 1992; Titley 1997).

Of particular concern in the context of this book is the role of primary health care and older people's relationships with their doctors. Andrews (1990) has observed that primary health care is important for older people in that it constitutes a critical point of entry to the health system. How access-ible that care is, what quality of service is provided and how people are treated in their encounters with their general practitioner (GP) will have a major impact on outcomes. This is especially important given that we know that in terms of consultation rates, older people (especially those aged 75 and over) are, with the under-fives, the highest consulters of doctors and that a sub-stantial majority come into contact with their GP or a member of the primary health care team at least once a year (Victor 1991; Kennie 1993). Higher pro-portions of women than men consult at all ages, although over a quarter of women aged 65 and over do not consult their doctor at all in any given year (Royal College of General Practitioners (RCGP) 1986). Marital status, class, housing tenure and ethnicity all compound this picture and show that widowed women, those from social classes IV and V, council house tenants and elderly Asian and African Caribbean people are among the highest con-sulters of doctors (Sidell 1995).

However, high consultation rates do not necessarily automatically translate into satisfaction with either services or professional responses. Feminist writers in Britain have been at the forefront of articulating the nature of the doctor–patient relationship (Foster 1995), although it has to be observed that the concerns of older women are still notable by their absence from much of the feminist literature (Bernard and Meade 1993). In the mid-1980s, Roberts (1985), drawing on evidence from medical textbooks and medical training, doctors' letters, and interviews with women and their doctors, revealed how the male-dominated medical profession regarded women differently from men in the medical literature and in practice. Other commentators have shown how 'many doctors still appear to regard women as innately more neurotic and prone to emotional instability than men' (Foster 1996: 107). As a consequence, because they expect female patients to behave in these ways, they will tend to treat them differently, prescribe them more mood alter-ing drugs, and offer insufficient and inadequate explanations for such com-plaints (Cooperstock 1979; Miles 1988; Ussher 1989). In combination with this sexist/patriarchal ideology, we must also be alert to both ageist and racist attitudes and practices, which have likewise been shown to influence people's satisfaction with the health care system in general, and doctors in particular (Ferraro 1987; Douglas 1992; Sidell 1992). For example, patient–doctor inter-actions are potentially difficult where cultural, racial and ethnic concerns such as language problems are concerned (Ahmad *et al.* 1989; Blakemore and Boneham 1993).

However, these kinds of issues do not, on the whole, get picked up by the large scale surveys to which we have already made reference and, again, we have to piece the evidence together from smaller scale qualitative studies (Sidell 1995; Beattie 1997a, 1997b; Bodie 1997). With regard to age, such qualitative data suggest that older people do not take the decision to visit their doctors lightly but that once they do, they may well be treated in an ageist manner or offered what seem to be inappropriate treatments (Bernard 1989; Sidell 1993). The manner in which information is both given and received is another area of dissatisfaction reported in some studies (Action for Health 1988; Wenger 1988; Sidell 1991). Older people feel that they are not listened to or given sufficient explanations about what the matter is with them, why they are given particular forms of treatment or what to expect. In the case of chronic illnesses this is especially important since effective management and treatment require a high level of patient involvement (Blakemore 1998).

Recent research concerning exercise advice and older people has also high-lighted the dangers of doctors' stereotyping according to chronological age, of being too quick to assume 'it's just your age' and often believing that it was too late for older people to derive benefit from such activity (Eadie *et al.* 1996; Stead *et al.* 1997). One graphic illustration of poor doctor–patient communi-cation comes from the Self Health Care in Old Age Project itself. It concerns an elderly woman who came into the Health Shop saying that she had been put on a low sodium diet by her GP. However, he had failed to tell her what this meant in practice – cutting down on salt – and she had been too anxious and too embarrassed to ask. Clearly, we still have much to learn about the interface between professional health providers and older people, points to which we shall return in subsequent chapters.

Conclusion

The discussions in this chapter strongly suggest that we need to reorient how we approach the subject of the health of older people. The information we have to date tends to focus on disease, illness and death, perpetuating the myths identified in the opening pages and reinforcing the negative assump-tions about the quality of health which can be expected in later life. The treat-ment meted out to older people, and the discriminatory and ageist attitudes they often encounter in their dealings with health and welfare services and personnel, exacerbate this situation. Consequently, instead of focusing on death and disease as much of the above discussion has done, we may in fact benefit from looking more closely at how older people keep themselves healthy and how this can be promoted and facilitated. This would move us away from the pathogenic biomedical model which emphasizes sickness and treatment, and more towards the salutogenic or health seeking framework proposed by Antonovsky (1984, 1987, 1996). Such a reorientation means that rather than trying to define people simplistically as healthy or diseased, we regard these terms at either end of a continuum. All of us, older and younger people alike, individually and collectively, can then be located some-where along this continuum.

The benefits of such a framework include its discouragement of the 'per-centage approach to assessing the health of older people' in favour of an emphasis on looking at how and why people cope; the turning on its head of the notion that older people are a high risk group thereby reinforcing the negative stereotype of them as disabled and diseased (Sidell 1997: 12–13); and a reaffirmation of the dynamic relationship which exists between people and their environment, including their relationships and social supports (Jones 1997b: 32). Indeed, such an approach underpins the Self Health Care in Old Age Project and lies at the heart of the health promotion and self health care activities detailed in succeeding chapters.

2

Promoting health in old age

Introduction

Having set the broad context for our examination of self health care in old age we move on, in this chapter, to explore the development of health promotion. In response to the growing interest and mounting activity around health and older people noted in Chapter 1, our prime concern here is with tracing the ways in which policy and practice have responded in the post-war years. Particular shifts are discernible over this time as we moved away from the early consensus about the NHS and began to question our reliance on purely medical approaches and interventions. There was also a growing recognition that the need for health care would always outstrip our ability to provide it (Blaxter 1996).

This recognition, together with a persistent thread of research on issues such as health inequalities, social class gradients and health, and poverty and health, has led to a much greater focus in recent years on the importance of understanding the social, political and environmental contexts of health, and on exploring preventive and health promoting approaches to health and well-being in later life. Parallels have been drawn between contemporary policy developments in this field and earlier approaches to public health, and this chapter therefore begins with a brief look at these antecedents. This leads into a discussion of healthy public policy and the new public health, before going on to consider the role of health promotion. The remainder of the chapter then concentrates specifically on health promotion and older people, examining evolving policy and practice in this area both during, and in the years since, the Beth Johnson Foundation's Self Health Care in Old Age Project was established in 1986.

The policy context

Contemporary health policy lays considerable emphasis on the creation of what has come to be called 'healthy public policy'. While there is debate in the literature about just what is meant by this term and how it relates to other approaches (Ashton and Seymour 1988; Pederson *et al.* 1988; Bunton 1993), we shall regard it for present purposes as an overarching approach to health. It draws on a variety of traditions, notably the Victorian public health movement in Britain, as well as on the wider development of social policy and social welfare during the twentieth century, and is closely integrated with more recent developments in health promotion, and what is now termed the 'new public health'. We shall briefly outline these developments in order to provide the reader with a sense of the context in which present day health promotion with older people has to operate.

Early approaches to public health can be traced back to the nineteenth century and attempts to improve the health of the populace – particularly in urban areas – through measures designed to counteract the virulent and widespread diseases of the time such as typhus, cholera and smallpox. Improvements in sanitation were the main means through which this was to be achieved, and advancements in civil engineering led to the development of effective sewage systems and improved water supplies. These measures were reinforced through the compulsory creation, across the UK, of medical officers of health and sanitary inspectors, and were backed up by a series of Public Health Acts from the 1840s onwards. In particular, the 1848 Act was notable for its articulation of the importance of public intervention in health, and its emphasis on a preventive, environmental model as opposed to a narrow medical one (Midwinter 1994). Towards the end of the nineteenth century, however, medical advances were moving on at such a pace that it was already possible to discern a shift towards a more curative approach in which hospitals and doctors were playing an increasingly prominent role.

In the twentieth century, cure and prevention became enduring twin themes in the pursuit of health. The old concerns about poor sanitation, and the problems attendant on rapid urbanization and overcrowding, have been succeeded by further measures designed to improve, for example, the air we breathe and the food we eat. Medical science too continued to bring an ever-widening range of infectious diseases under control, with forms of both prevention (through immunization and vaccination) and treatment being addressed. At the same time, public health as it had originally been understood and enacted was increasingly regarded as having reached the limits of its success and its status declined in polar opposition to the rise of curative medicine (Jones 1997a). Public health medicine, with its emphasis on prevention, tended to become marginalized until, as we shall see below, it was revived again in the mid-1980s under the guise of the new public health.

No less important to health, but not often associated with the traditional public health movement, have been improvements and legislation in associated areas such as housing, working conditions, poverty, employment and transportation. These broader dimensions of social welfare have also had considerable influence on the development of healthy public policy. During the twentieth century, they came to assume greater or lesser relevance to health as certain concerns superseded others, and as different political ideologies and beliefs came to the fore. Indeed, coming out of this longer social welfare tradition, it could be argued that it was a recognition of the close interaction between health and these aspects, that was one of the driving forces behind the creation of the welfare state.

In the wake of the creation of the NHS in 1948, it was hardly surprising then that 'the provision of universally available medical care was seen as a vital part of policy for improving health standards throughout society' (Blane *et al.* 1996: 2). Medical care, free to all at the point of delivery, was closely linked with other welfare measures and reforms to provide a safety net for the entire populace: Beveridge's much vaunted 'cradle-to-grave' insurance against sickness, poverty and unemployment. However, it is also important to remember that when the NHS was established in 1948, the socio-demographic, economic and political contexts were very different from those which pertain at the present time. It was set up against a background of decades of incomplete health insurance cover and inadequate services. Many people had been unable to pay for the services and treatments they needed, and it was only with the Beveridge Report of 1942 that proposals were brought forward for the reform of the social service system and the creation of a national health service. The 1946 Act had a difficult passage through the legislative system because of its radical proposals to transform what had been an inadequate and muddled patchwork of health care provision (Klein 1989). However, it did eventually succeed in rationalizing the administrative structures and was the first health system in the western world to extend free medical treatment and health care to the entire population.

Despite the principles of free and universal health and medical care, expectations that the health of the nation would improve dramatically and thereby lead to a reduction in the need for health care, very soon proved wrong (Manning 1994). In effect, the medical aspects of these policy reforms have become ever more divorced from other welfare and preventive services, despite Beveridge's original desire to have a national health service which would tackle both prevention and cure through medical treatment. Moreover, commentators on the reforms have shown how policy in the decades since the establishment of the NHS has been dogged by the continuing conflicts between the NHS as a political ideal, and the practicalities of actually delivering that care to the population as ill health, like poverty, refused to disappear and the inequalities and social class differences, rather than narrowing, became ever more apparent (Midwinter 1994; Klein 1995; Blane *et al.* 1996; Taylor and Field 1997).

By the 1960s, MacDonald (1998: 21) contends that despite all these public health measures and policy reforms, people had in fact stopped becoming healthier and a new direction and response was called for. This realization contributed, as Ashton and Seymour (1988) have noted, to a marked shift of emphasis away from the 'public' and towards the 'private' in health matters. Health, in contrast to illness and disease, came to be seen more and more as an issue for individuals in comparative isolation from social or environmental determinants. It also contributed, as Blane and his colleagues (1996: 4) have noted, 'to the belief that social policy was no longer such an important part of preventive health policy'.

Against a background of global economic recession, continuing domestic inflation and the oil crisis of the early 1970s, Britain, as Klein (1989: 171) has famously observed, 'rediscovered prevention'. Initially, however, prevention was couched very much within an individual behaviour change model which simply reinforced the public–private split and left unchallenged the structural and environmental aspects of ill health. At this time too, the state of the NHS was being much debated, and a Royal Commission was established to examine its future prospects in detail. Alongside this, the ideology of the benefits of community care over institutional care was also rapidly becoming 'an article of faith' (Dalley 1998: 26). Thus, with the arrival of the Thatcher government in 1979, the stage was well and truly set for major changes in the provision of health care, driven by a political ideology which espoused individual responsibility and which was wedded to steering through radical structural changes.

Healthy public policy, the new public health and health promotion

The need for a new direction and response is now encapsulated in the development of what is termed 'healthy public policy'. Healthy public policy can be viewed as a concept, as a goal and as an ideology. Its articulation as a concept encompasses a recognition that policies other than health influence choices, and that in order to achieve the goal of healthy public policy, we have to incorporate a range of integrated policy changes together with greater public participation in health (WHO 1985; Popay *et al.* 1993). The notion of 'health for all by the year 2000' came to symbolize this orientation and found expression in a series of documents and strategies stretching back to 1977, the year that this call was first adopted by the World Health Organization (1977). Since then, the goal of healthy public policy has been encapsulated in various proposals and target setting exercises beginning with the Alma Ata declaration in 1978 and extending on through the 1980s and 1990s at both national and international levels (WHO 1978, 1985). Alongside this, other wider connections have been made notably, as Jones (1997a: 93) observes, 'the linking together of healthy public policy and supportive environments'. Here, environmental concerns and environmental protection feature strongly, with the idea of communities working together to improve health being a key strategy. Moreover, following the election of a Labour government in May 1997, Britain saw the appointment of its first ever Minister for Public Health in the person of Tessa Jowell. One of her first actions was, interestingly, to commission an inquiry into inequalities in health which updated the 1980 Black Report (Townsend and Davidson 1986) and reaffirmed, yet again, the major impact which poverty has on health.

The new public health approach which has thus emerged brings together the concept of healthy public policy, with health promotion policies and approaches. The 'newness' of the new public health has to do both with its focus, and its concerns. It has, as its focus, an emphasis on creating and sustaining a healthy society in contrast with the 'old' public health which historically focused on sustaining a medically oriented notion of health. Then, the primary goal of public health medicine was to improve medical care of ill people and thereby improve the health of the general populace. Now, the goal is broader and, drawing on its Victorian legacy, the new public health incorporates a holistic view, arguing that health cannot be adequately understood without taking into account the wider environments in which we live out our lives. The new public health perspective is characterized by a concern with social and psychological, as well as physical factors, concerns which extend from the local to the global and which explicitly seek to address socio-economic determinants of health (Ashton and Seymour 1988; Public Health Alliance (PHA) 1994; MacDonald 1998). 'Environment' and 'lifestyle' are key notions in this perspective, and both are seen as legitimate areas for intervention in order to improve people's health (Davison and Davey Smith 1995).

Inextricably linked with the new public health has been the emergence of health promotion, both as a policy arena and as a field of practice. For some, the new public health directly influences, and acts through health promotion, such that 'the principles and content of modern health promotion . . . are identical to those of the new public health' (MacDonald 1998: 28). Others draw distinctions between healthy public policy, the new public health and health promotion, in which health promotion is regarded as quite specific kinds of programmes, activities and policies (Bunton 1993). In policy terms, we can date health promotion back to the early 1970s and to the work, in Canada, of Marc Lalonde. As the then Canadian Minister for Health and Welfare, he was responsible for the publication of the Lalonde Report (1974) which proposed that health was influenced by a number of 'fields': biology, lifestyle, environment and the organization of health care. The report also discussed the relative importance of, and links between, the individual and society. It thus drew attention to a range of important influences on health, and began a process of critically questioning our reliance on a purely biomedical model in which the dominance of the medical profession was taken for granted. While regarded as a milestone in health promotion policy, it did not transform our views overnight, although it did signal that changes were afoot (Kelly and Charlton 1995; MacDonald 1998).

This change of perspective can subsequently be traced through the work of the World Health Organization, and its continuing influence on national and international strategies for health. The famous Alma Ata declaration of 1978 reasserted the view that health was about much more than just the absence of disease or infirmity and, by the end of the decade, the 32 WHO member states had accepted targets and indicators in support of the proposals contained in the Health for All by the Year 2000 strategy (Macfadyen 1985; Parish 1995). The UK agreed to monitor progress towards the indicators contained in the strategy, but did not itself establish one. It had in fact begun to stimulate its own debate a year earlier with the publication of a discussion document entitled *Prevention and Health: Everybody's Business* (Department of Health and Social Security (DHSS) 1976). Like the Alma Ata declaration, this document asked questions about the appropriate role of government in health matters, and it also drew attention to geographical and social class variations in health. Unlike the declaration, however, it was on less sure ground when it came to discussing whose responsibility health might be, and what might influence it. Nonetheless, it was the first in a long line of government papers and documents which kept health and health promotion issues high on the domestic agenda in Britain during the 1980s.

The dawn of the 1980s also witnessed the emergence of the notion of 'health promotion', although it was 1986 before there was any attempt to try to reach a consensus about what the term might mean (MacDonald 1998). In 1980, the WHO Regional Office for Europe was involved in developing a four-year programme of health education amidst a growing recognition that health education in and of itself was insufficient to promote the necessary changes at national levels. This led to the creation of a parallel health pro-motion programme with its own budget and staff which began work in 1984 and which concentrated on five main issues (Parish 1995):

1 Improving access to health.
2 Developing an environment conducive to health.
3 Strengthening social networks and social supports.
4 Promoting positive health behaviour and appropriate coping strategies.
5 Increasing knowledge and disseminating information.

(Parish 1995: 22)

This programme was also important for drawing attention to a number of concerns which have been reiterated down the years. In particular, it cau-tioned against the dangers of professionalization and of health promotion becoming too prescriptive; of individualizing health and health promotion programmes to such an extent that they help create and reinforce a victim-blaming culture; and of the possibilities of exacerbating inequities unless education, information and awareness raising was also accompanied by increasing people's control (Kalache *et al.* 1988).

In Britain, the then Health Education Council was beginning to be active in this area and (as we shall see below) was instrumental in developing health promotion with and for older people. In Canada, the 1986 Ottawa Charter for Health Promotion marked a further important development in that for the first time, health promotion was seen as a framework for health which extended beyond formal health care and was a societal, as well as an indi-vidual responsibility. The Charter, introduced by Jake Epp, Minister of National Health and Welfare, drew attention to what it regarded as a number of prerequisites for health: peace, shelter, education, food, income, a stable ecosystem, sustainable resources, social justice and equity. In order to achieve the WHO goal of health for all and to build healthy public policy, the Ottawa Charter set out a framework which echoed the concerns of the WHO's health promotion programme, and also involved five elements:

1 Strengthening community action.
2 Developing personal skills.
3 Enabling, mediating and advocating.
4 Creating supportive environments.
5 Reorienting health services.

Together, these elements encapsulated a number of challenges which had –

and still have – a particular relevance for health promotion work with older people. These included the need to think about how one might enhance people's capacity to cope with chronic disease and disability and with emotional pain; how to shift the emphasis away from professionals and towards individuals and communities; ways of addressing poverty, social justice and inequities; the need to reorient services towards primary health care and preventive activities; and the importance of developing cross-sectoral and inter-agency working (McClymont *et al.* 1991; Granville 1996; MacDonald 1998). Launched at the annual conference of the Canadian Public Health Association, the Ottawa Charter gave a real impetus to the development of comprehensive national health strategies as envisaged by the WHO. Moreover, Canada has also had, since the late 1980s, a Seniors' Strategy as an integral part of their policies. Here, the emphasis is clearly on collective responsibility and community participation (Killoran *et al.* 1997). Since 1994, this has underpinned what is now a very much larger initiative designed to address the challenges of an ageing population. Their 'National Framework on Aging' is a multi-perspective model with an explicit and common inter-sectoral approach, and a focus on the determinants of health.

However, it was to be another five years after the Ottawa Charter before a health strategy for England was published. Commentators on the domestic scene argue that such a slow response was due primarily to a lack of political will and to an unwillingness to accept that government had a strategic role to play in the development of healthy public policy (Parish 1995). Wales, by contrast, was somewhat more forward thinking in this area (Jones 1997a). Although the development and evolution of the UK strategies are all different, in essence, all the most recent documentation is target-oriented: they identify a series of issues to be addressed such as smoking, and establish a suite of measures to be taken against which progress can be assessed. In England, the 1991 consultative Green Paper first set out a series of Health of the Nation targets which, after extensive discussion, was issued a year later as *The Health of the Nation: A Strategy for Health in England* (Department of Health (DoH) 1992). This strategy was aimed at the entire population and hoped for significant improvements in morbidity and mortality around a series of key areas: coronary heart disease and strokes; cancers; accidental injury; mental illness; and HIV/AIDS and sexual health (oral health was to be added later in 1995).

Not surprisingly, the strategy was both welcomed and criticized. It was welcomed for at long last putting health promotion policy on the national agenda (Ewles 1996), for recognizing that government had a role to play in promoting the health of the populace, and for acknowledging that health issues need to be addressed in a variety of settings and environments (Jones 1997a). However, it was also the subject of considerable criticism: for its narrow individual behavioural view of health and its disease focus; its reliance on a traditional model of preventive health education at the expense of the more radical WHO philosophy (Tones and Tilford 1994); its sidestepping of issues related to socio-economic factors, to poverty, inequality and the political dimensions of health (Benzeval *et al.* 1995; Nettleton and Bunton 1995); and, of particular importance to the concerns of this book, its failure to include the health of older people (or rehabilitation services) as a key area (Dalley *et al.*

1996; MacDonald 1998). The emphasis on reducing premature death and the specification of age limits which, for example, exclude people aged 75 and over from the coronary heart disease and stroke targets, has led to the pertinent observation that 'This policy implies that improving health is less worthwhile for older people than for younger and is therefore ageist' (Ginn *et al.* 1997: 7). Moreover, although organizations like the British Geriatrics Society (1993) have commented on the key areas as they apply to older people, we are still left with the realization that, as Killoran and her colleagues (1997) have noted:

> The strategy represents a missed opportunity to develop a systematic and coherent approach to reducing the burden of illness in the older population. The strategy leaves a lacuna which remains to be filled. To fill this lacuna, moreover, would require an explicit and articulated commitment to the pursuit of a goal over and above the extension of life expectancy.
> (Killoran *et al.* 1997: 17)

That this opportunity has been missed at a national policy level is all the more lamentable, given the range of initiatives and practical developments and programmes that were operating during the 1980s.

Health promotion and older people: national initiatives

Although recent national policy may downplay the importance of health promotion for older people, the 1980s was in fact a decade of considerable activity in this area. At the time the Beth Johnson Foundation began to develop its health and related activities in the first half of the 1980s (see Chapter 5), the Health Education Council (as it was then known, later renamed the Health Education Authority) was putting together plans for what was to become the Health in Old Age Programme. This programme followed extensive consultation with a variety of organizations and individuals (Huntington 1985), a number of commissioned research projects examining aspects of health education and older people (see, for example, Phillipson and Strang 1984; Groombridge 1988; Coleman and Chira 1991), and the mounting of two collaborative national seminars (Glendenning 1985, 1986). In respect of the consultation exercise, Huntington (1985: 105–6) details several major themes which emerged from the responses, and which illustrate just how embryonic our understanding and knowledge about health promotion and older people was at that time. The themes were as follows:

- The need to raise expectations of health in old age among the total population.
- The key role of professional health workers.
- The importance of voluntary carers and the need for recognition of both their contribution and their needs.
- The need to recognize and evaluate the extensive work already underway.
- The need to recognize that different groups of elderly people have different needs, to consult them about the services they require, and to plan accordingly.
- The importance of cooperation between different groups working with elderly people, and between professionals and volunteers.
- The need for appropriate and well-presented educational materials.

In addition to these general themes, respondents to the consultation exercise made detailed recommendations about the specific topics which might be considered under a national health education programme. These topics included:

- back pain
- bereavement
- continence
- deafness
- dementia
- dental health needs
- diet and nutrition
- emotional health
- exercise, physical activity and sport in old age
- first aid
- foot care
- hypothermia
- mental health
- problems with drugs/understanding medication
- self health care
- smoking
- unsteadiness, falls and accident prevention.

The special needs of minority ethnic elders, of older women and of older men separately, of people coming up to retirement, and of informal carers, were also highlighted as important issues to be addressed. The need to consider the attitudes of those who work in this field, and to develop opportunities for inter-professional training was also regarded as important in order for the programme to be able to contribute to the reduction of the negative stereotypes and stigma associated with old age.

Funded by the then Department of Health and Social Security (DHSS) and dubbed the Health in Old Age Programme, the five-year plan was eventually launched in the spring of 1985, and aimed at adults over the age of 50. As the first British programme of its kind, its overall aim was 'to enhance the potential of older people to live independent healthy lives in the community, and to enable those who are approaching retirement to develop self care skills for the future' (Health Education Council (HEC) 1985: 2). The programme consisted of four main strategies, organized into three distinct, but overlapping, phases. The strategies were as follows:

- *Education activities* – both with older people themselves, and in respect of training and development of professionals and of informal carers.
- *Information and materials* – for older people themselves, for professionals and for carers.
- *Public awareness campaigns* – to support the first two strategies, and with a commitment to encouraging complementary activity at a local level coordinated with the HEC's initiatives.
- *Collaboration* – with existing groups, especially national, voluntary and statutory organizations and professional bodies.

The first, two-year phase of the programme was directed at development and dissemination activities: collating and disseminating the results of existing work and examples of good practice. To this end the HEC, together with Age Concern England, coordinated the Age Well campaign and produced the Age Well Ideas Packs consisting of details of health initiatives across the UK (HEC/Age Concern 1985; Health Education Authority (HEA)/Age Concern 1988). Over subsequent years, efforts were to be directed towards increasing public awareness of the need to promote a more positive approach to health in old age, and at giving continued encouragement to the development of more self-sustaining activities at the local level.

In reality, activity other than the Age Well campaign was very low key and very localized. The scale of it was fairly modest, especially when set alongside the kinds of activity and expenditure devoted to curative, hospital-based services. It did, though, contribute to the emerging consciousness among organizations which worked with older people, of the tremendous need and potential to enhance the health and well-being of older adults. At this time too, the Sports Council was involved in initiating sport and leisure activities for older people. In 1982, it produced a report entitled *Sport in the Community: The Next Ten Years*, which identified people aged 45 to 59 as one of its target groups. During its ensuing five-year programme (1983–7) the aim was to attract nearly a quarter of a million more women and men into physical activity. The following year, the Sports Council instigated its 'Fifty Plus – And All To Play For' Campaign, with fifty separate launches around the UK. The emphasis here was on a light-hearted approach to physical activity, stressing the fun and enjoyment that could be derived in addition to the health benefits.

These programmes were followed in the late 1980s and 1990s by other reports and initiatives. In 1988, an attempt was made to respond directly to the Ottawa Charter through a joint working party set up by the London School of Tropical Medicine and Hygiene, the Age Concern Institute of Gerontology and the King's Fund Institute (Kalache *et al.* 1988). The short report produced by this group was important for drawing attention to two key issues. First, in a clear echo of the World Health Organization, it stated that health promotion and the health of older people was not simply a matter for the Department of Health, and that health promotion and ageing should be put 'onto the agendas of other departments and agencies in the fields of transport, education, environment and housing to ensure that policy initiatives do not run counter to the notion of positive health' (Kalache *et al.* 1988: 35). Second, it drew attention to the chronic lack of research and evaluation about health promotion and older people, an issue which is taken up in later chapters.

In the 1990s, and following the publication of the Health of the Nation strategy, two further initiatives have begun to bring the health promotion needs of older people onto national and local agendas again. The original Age Well campaign of the 1980s has developed into Ageing Well UK, a programme which was designed specifically to maximize the potential of older people as a health resource for their peers (Ashton 1995). This three-year programme (1994–7) drew not only on Age Concern England's own work but also very considerably on the peer health counselling developments initiated by the Beth Johnson Foundation in the 1980s (Bernard 1993). Twelve projects, all using senior health mentors, have been established around the UK and were evaluated by the Age Concern Institute. In addition, the Health Education Authority launched a new three-year programme in 1996 directed at improving physical activity among adults, with people aged 50-plus being a special target group. The Active for Life campaign is reminiscent of the 1980s' 'Sport For All' and 'Fifty Plus – And All To Play For' ventures and illustrates, yet again, how far we still have to go in developing national policies and activities which will truly and comprehensively address the health of older people. While we can point to a whole gamut of initiatives and projects during the 1980s and 1990s, we are still some way from developing a framework for both action and research, a point to which we shall return in the concluding chapter.

For the present, however, this discussion of the policy context and of the development of particular initiatives begs the important question of what health promotion with and for older people really is. In the last section of this chapter, we therefore turn our attention to this issue and examine the nature of health promotion and its defining characteristics.

Health promotion and older people

Like health promotion generally, health promotion with older people can be regarded as having a number of related activities and components. Health promotion is a much debated and contested concept, but is usually considered to have a health protection strand, a preventive strand and an educative strand (Tannahill 1985). These in turn can be linked to the policy issues discussed above which are required to develop healthy public policy. The *health protection* strand has perhaps the most obvious link and can be traced back to traditional public health approaches. In essence, this reiterates the importance of measures enacted to protect the health of the populace and would include things such as bans on smoking in public places and car seat-belt laws.

Health prevention by contrast would include specific measures to address ill health, reduce disease and conserve, rather than actively improve, health. We commonly identify three levels of prevention: primary – which aims to prevent people getting a disease or disorder by using measures such as vaccinating older people against flu; secondary – which tries to detect a condition in its early stages and might, for example, include screening of women with known risk factors for osteoporosis (Granville 1996); and tertiary – which consists of active treatment of a particular condition or illness in order to reduce its effects (Ashton and Seymour 1993). As Sidell (1995: 162) argues, highly successful primary and secondary prevention would eventually lead to the kind of scenario depicted by Fries in his compression of morbidity thesis discussed in Chapter 1. Tertiary prevention, meanwhile, is of particular relevance to older people since treatment of chronic conditions in particular would do much to improve their quality of life and well-being.

Health education in turn is characterized by an emphasis on information and advice giving, in which the aim is to educate both individuals and the wider community. This suggests that education is a one-way process but, as health promotion itself has developed, a more radical view of the role of health education has emerged. The tendency now is to conceptualize it less as a top-down approach but more as a two-way process which is both contextualized and in which issues such as attitudes and values become legitimate areas for exploration and intervention (Tones 1996). Health education has in fact shifted in meaning over time. This has, in turn, led to the formulation of models which attempt to delineate the various approaches to, and dimensions of, health promotion practice (for a discussion of these models, see Jones and Naidoo 1997: ch. 5). A particular feature of these shifts in meaning is that the notion of 'empowerment' has become key to health promotion policy and practice. Moreover, since empowerment has been a fundamental underpinning of the work of the Beth Johnson Foundation, it is itself an issue we consider further below.

To these three health promotion strands of protection, prevention and education, we can also add a fourth: *health preservation*. For older people in particular, there is a growing recognition that achieving optimal levels of functioning is vitally important. Incorporating dimensions which are explicitly about functioning as opposed to disability, would take us beyond the mortality and morbidity measures discussed in Chapter 1 and, if integrated into health promotion programmes could help us reorient how we think about health and older people along Antonovsky's (1996) salutogenic (health seeking) as opposed to pathogenic (illness) lines (Killoran *et al.* 1997).

Health promotion, older people and empowerment

Health promotion work with older people has taken some considerable time to be perceived as a legitimate area of concern and attention in Britain. Although there have been attempts to develop activity at local levels since the mid-1980s, this has not been mirrored at a policy level. Local level activity around health promotion and health education, including the Beth Johnson Foundation's own developments, has employed a range of approaches. Our own work in particular was influenced by a number of strands. Importantly, this has included perspectives from education, traceable back to the seminal work of Paulo Freire (1972, 1973, 1974) on emancipatory education and critical consciousness raising, and on through wider developments in the educational gerontology field (Glendenning and Percy 1990); perspectives from, and a commitment to, the tenets and ways of working associated with a community development approach and the self-help movement (Twelvetrees 1982; Richardson and Goodman 1983); and perspectives from some of what were, at the time, the more radical critiques of health education propounded by authors such as Tones (1981, 1983) and Beattie (1984). What is common to all these strands and perspectives is the notion of *empowerment*.

Empowerment, like health promotion itself, is a much used and abused concept. It is therefore important here to consider how we use and understand the term, given the central concern of this book with the development of health promotion generally, and self health care in old age specifically. In terms of definitions, empowerment can be variously understood as an ideal or ethos, as a goal, as a skill, as a process or set of processes, and as an outcome or outcomes (Gutierrez 1990; Stevenson and Parsloe 1993; Cox and Parsons 1994; Thursz *et al.* 1995; MacDonald 1998). As we have seen above, the mid-1980s was a time when health promotion was emerging onto the national and international scene and, as Beeker and her colleagues note (1998: 832), it had 'empowerment as its ideological center and citizen participation as its primary strategy'. In addition to its close association with education, health promotion and community development work, empowerment has also been central to the development of the discipline of community psychology (Rappaport 1981, 1984, 1987; Rappaport *et al.* 1984), a key element of much social work activity (Staples 1990; Cheetham *et al.* 1992; Cox and Parsons 1994; Braye and Preston-Shoot 1995; Browne 1995) and an underlying feature of feminist theorizing and analysis stretching back some 40 years to the work of Hannah Arendt (1958; see also Browne 1998). Since the mid-1990s it has also spawned a literature on 'empowerment evaluation' derived originally from models of community health and development (Fawcett *et al.* 1994, 1995; Fawcett 1995; Fetterman *et al.* 1996). Yet, despite this plethora of work, empowerment remains an ill-defined and much contested concept (Barnes and Warren 1999). This in turn suggests that empowerment may be a very difficult term to try and measure and, indeed, this was an issue with which we too struggled in the Self Health Care in Old Age Project.

One way forward is to try to unpack further what we might mean by empowerment. As a first step, we have to recognize that empowerment can operate at different levels: individual, organizational and community. At an individual level, empowerment is essentially about the acquisition of particular skills and/or a change to the ways one thinks about oneself. Much has been written about individual empowerment and how it is linked with taking control over one's life and one's destiny (Adams 1990; Meade and Carter 1990; Staples 1990; Zimmerman 1995). Given our present concerns, it is also pertinent to note here that some writers link individual empowerment with a recognition that it needs to build on existing skills and competencies (Rappaport *et al.* 1984), and that a raising of people's consciousness and confidence will lead to increased participation (Rissel 1994), and an enhanced ability to weigh up and make appropriate choices (Stevenson and Parsloe 1993). Individual empowerment in this sense is an overwhelmingly positive and dynamic notion, concerned with growth and personal development (Staples 1990). It is also a means by which, in health promotion terms, 'individual people are encouraged to assert their own autonomy and self esteem sufficiently to be able to identify their own health agenda, rather than being told what to do or what is "good for your health"' (MacDonald 1998: 8).

In the realms of organizational empowerment, we move on to a different set of understandings and issues which lead us to begin to question the relationship between individuals and structures. While it may be possible to become empowered in and of oneself, organizational cultures are important either as facilitators or impediments to those processes, both for staff who work within them and for those with whom staff work – in our case, older people. We are dealing here both with the attitudes and orientations of professionals, be they health and social service personnel, or be they voluntary sector workers and volunteers; and with organizational frameworks. It is not, for example, very empowering if a health worker has supported and facilitated an elderly patient to speak out about the treatment she receives in a nursing home, if that home's structure and culture has no means to hear those concerns and is resistant to being criticized, however constructively. In the context of a project which examined the implementation of the NHS and Community Care Act 1990, Stevenson and Parsloe (1993) encapsulate this dilemma thus:

> As users and carers experience more power, what was formerly accept-able will be criticised. The same is true for staff. Empowerment is an evolving process and has no clear end point, which may explain the reluctance and fear with which it is sometimes regarded.
>
> (Stevenson and Parslow 1993: 10)

The reluctance and fear that these authors note is less in evidence when we look at community level empowerment. Indeed, empowerment through community mobilization and support has been a cornerstone of community development approaches, with community workers acting as go-betweens and as facilitators (Craig and Mayo 1995; Sidell 1997). In the health pro-motion arena this is a well established approach built around a recognition that community empowerment will come about only through the active par-ticipation of people in both the planning and implementation of change, and through assisting communities to access and use a range of resources most effectively – what has been termed 'community capacity-building' in the literature (Croft and Beresford 1992; Beeker *et al.* 1998).

At whichever level one considers empowerment, there are two fundamental issues to be considered further. First, there is the issue of power itself: what it is, who has it and how it is distributed. The second issue concerns the relation-ship between individuals: the client/patient and the professional; the elderly person and the younger volunteer; the front line worker and the manager.

Power is a very evocative word. Dictionary definitions stress the ways in which power is about having the ability, strength or position of authority to determine, control or influence someone or something. Meanwhile, a thes-aurus will list synonyms such as ascendancy, authority, domination, force, leverage, command and strength and its antonyms as impotence, infirmity, subservience and weakness. Incorporating such meanings into the notion of empowerment itself suggests, in turn, that power is in some ways a finite capacity: that there is a certain amount of it to go round and that what is key is how it is divided up and who has it. In order to become empowered within this framework, there is a suggestion that power itself has either to be given to, given up by, or taken from someone else or some other group of people. Conventionally, empowerment has therefore come to be viewed in very indi-vidualistic terms. It is also no surprise that we still speak and write in terms of the *dominance* of the biomedical model in relation to health issues, ageing and older people – language which itself conveys the inherent inequalities of power. MacDonald (1998: 10) has suggested that it might be more appropri-ate to refer to the act of conferring power on a patient or client by someone in authority as *impowerment*, reserving empowerment for 'the cultivation of a person's self esteem to such a degree that they assume power over some aspect of their life, without reference to higher authority'.

Feminist critiques of power, on the other hand, view it much more in terms of a process than a finite 'thing' that can be parcelled out, regarding it more as a creative force or energy (Browne 1998). Reorienting how we think about power in this way and stressing, as Minkler (1996) does, that power is about social relatedness, community good and interdependence as opposed to individual good and independence, has special relevance and importance for older people and those of us who work in this arena. It has, for example, been argued that for older women in particular, it offers the possibility of helping us to look more positively and constructively at the diversity, complexity and commonalities in their lives, instead of in simplistic dualisms (such as the powerless versus the powerful) and through a predominantly pathological lens (Browne 1998). In this sense then power and by extension empowerment are clearly very much about the nature of the relationships which exist between people.

At the heart of these relationships is the closely associated issue of knowledge, and particularly professional as opposed to lay knowledge. By laying claim to and maintaining a particular body of knowledge, health and welfare professionals are in a tremendously powerful position. In the current struggles to try to counteract negative images of ageing and the ways in which services respond to older people, empowerment has been seized upon as a means to address some of these problems. However, important cautions and warnings have been sounded by many authors. First, it has been strongly argued that empowerment of older people is not the same thing as consultation by professionals (Walker and Warren 1996). Yet, 'consumer consultation' along with 'user empowerment' have become buzz phrases in the wake of much health and social welfare legislation of the 1990s. Second, others have questioned whether professionals can ever truly empower clients and patients when they are, by definition, in an unequal power relationship to begin with. As Stevenson and Cooper (1996: 149) have cogently observed: 'giving power to others is implicitly a power play, and it can be argued that the client who is the passive recipient of power, therefore, is not actually empowered'.

Furthermore, professional attempts to empower clients or patients are considered by some simply as a crude means of maintaining control (Grace 1991). These kinds of critiques show that there is clearly an onus on the professional to learn to be reflexive both about their own role and about their position in respect of their relationship with clients and patients. Indeed, Stevenson and Parsloe (1993: 10–11) go so far as to suggest that empowerment of staff is just as important as the empowerment of users and carers, and that this 'demands not just new ways of working but also changes in the attitudes which underlie that work ... It requires an active worker ready to share ideas and thoughts and to ensure that the other has the advantage of hearing different points of view'. Such changes in attitudes and in working practices have to go hand-in-hand with any attempt at empowerment. Indeed, it is said that empowerment can really work only 'by raising awareness of the ways in which power is exerted' (Sidell 1997: 51) and this applies equally to all those involved in a given relationship.

Finally, where we are engaged in trying to empower others, it has been suggested that not only do we need to be reflexive and aware of how power operates and manifests itself in certain contexts, but also we need to function according to certain principles and values. Croft and Beresford (1990, 1992, 1995) have written extensively around these issues in the context of user participation and citizen involvement, while Barnes and Walker (1996) list eight key principles which they believe should underlie attempts at empowerment.

These principles encapsulate many of the points made above and are salutary reminders of the need to think critically about what we mean by the term and how we operationalize it in our everyday practices. The eight principles are as follows:

1 Empowerment should enable personal development as well as increasing influence over services.
2 Empowerment should involve increasing people's abilities to take control of their lives as a whole, not just increase their influence over services.
3 Empowerment of one person should not result in the exploitation of others: either family members or paid carers.
4 Empowerment should not be viewed as a zero-sum: a partnership model should provide benefits to both parties.
5 Empowerment must be reinforced at all levels within service systems.
6 Empowerment of those who use services does not remove the responsibilities of those who produce them.
7 Empowerment is not an alternative to adequate resourcing of services.
8 Empowerment should be a collective as well as an individual process; without this people will become increasingly assertive in competition with each other.

This kind of principled approach is essentially about the need to work in partnership. Moreover, as Minkler (1996: 474) argues, and as we go on to demonstrate in Chapter 4, 'an empowering approach to working in partnership with older people would start where the people are'.

Conclusion

We have seen in this chapter how policy and practice around health promotion and older people has waxed and waned. The argument has been twofold. First, although promoting healthy lifestyles – healthy public policy in the current jargon – had been an underlying thread of policy over the twentieth century, older people have rarely, if ever, featured as a legitimate concern at least until the 1990s. Second, despite this lack of overt policy attention, the demographic, social, economic and political transformations which we have experienced since the 1960s, have contributed to grassroots initiatives and practical developments which have gradually been helping us to rethink some of the ways we approach health in later life. We are left then with the issue of not whether health promotion and empowerment are relevant to older people – they most certainly are – but how these are best translated into activities and practices which are accessible and beneficial. These are the major concerns of the ensuing chapters and we turn first to consider the place of self health care in the overall health promotion framework.

3

Perspectives on self health care

Introduction

Having outlined some of the forces that have led to a growing interest and concern with the health of older people, the purpose of this chapter is to introduce readers to the concept of self health care, and to examine its relationship with other allied notions such as self-help, self-care and empowerment. As with any new and emerging field of study and practice, one of the early problems we face is in trying to clarify what exactly we mean when we write and talk about the ideas associated with self health care. It cannot be automatically assumed that there are shared understandings and, as we shall see, there are a great many nuances of definition.

Allied to definitional and conceptual issues, we have also to consider the state of research on this topic. A major contention of this chapter is that existing research is, to say the least, patchy and fragmented. This is not to say that nothing has been done because, even in the late 1970s, the literature was already being described as having 'reached monumental proportions' (Butler *et al.* 1979: 112). Indeed, to synthesize all of it would be an impossible task within the scope of a text such as this. A further aim of the chapter is therefore to provide the reader with some indication of the kinds of research which have been carried out since self-care first appeared in the literature in the 1970s (Holstein 1986).

Through this examination of definitional, conceptual and research issues, it should become evident that older people, perhaps contrary to popular belief, are in fact well used to taking care of their own health. Policy and practice though, organized predominantly around a biomedical model emphasizing disease, disability and the associated problems of old age, has failed as yet to take adequate cognizance of this. The chapter therefore concludes with a suggestion that the time is now right to reorient our responses and policies around a salutogenic approach which emphasizes self-empowered health behaviour. This would acknowledge the experiences and skills of older people themselves, while supporting them within a broader health promotion framework which provides opportunities for improved information, enhanced self-health skills, and better access to health-related resources.

Defining what we mean

In his preface to the seminal volume *Self-Care and Health in Old Age* (Dean *et al.* 1986), Raymond Illsley writes about the distrust and suspicion which he originally harboured towards, in this instance, the notion of self-care. This suspicion was twofold. On the one hand, he felt that the concept was 'fuzzy', while on the other it was downright dangerous, in the sense that it could easily be hijacked into service by an anti-welfare, cost-cutting government and used as a further means to limit necessary resources and services. Its development, though, outgrew Illsley's suspicions, and his observations about the ways in which concepts and ideas evolve are highly pertinent to our discussions in this chapter. He writes:

> I suspect that many deep-rooted social movements start as fuzzy concepts because they represent an early, groping awareness of something that is wrong and something that needs to be done.
>
> If they are innovative and, particularly, if they challenge current values and practice, an accurate terminology may not exist and terms may be overladen with unwanted meanings from the past.
>
> (Illsley 1986)

While it is perhaps somewhat premature to claim that self-care/self health care is a 'deep-rooted social movement', the point about the lack of 'an accurate terminology' and associated terms is crucial. The growing body of research in Europe and North America addressing the theory, methodology and practice of self-care (*Social Science and Medicine* – special issue 29(2) 1989; *Generations* – special issue 17(3) 1993) is testimony to the growing interest in these ideas. Yet, as we shall see, conceptual clarity is still an issue for discussion and debate.

In what follows, I review a variety of terms in order to try to map out more precisely what it is that we are talking about. Kickbusch and Hatch (1983: 6) have suggested that it is possible to identify a self-help movement or continuum in relation to health care, 'which ranges from individual involvement in self care to possibly large scale action on the part of self help organisations'. This continuum provides a useful framework for exploring the range of inter-related concepts with which we are concerned. It also provided the basis, during the 1980s, for the work of the World Health Organization's Regional Office for Europe on *Self Help and Health in Europe* (Hatch and Kickbusch 1983). The continuum includes:

- *self-help* – which in turn encompasses self-help groups, self-help organizations and alternative care;
- *lay and volunteer care*;
- *self-care and self health care*.

Each of these will be discussed in turn, but what is immediately evident from this list is that the variety of health care which we are considering here emphasizes the social, not simply the medical aspects of health. Such a social model encompasses individual involvement in health maintenance behaviours as well as larger scale action by groups and organizations. It also highlights the need to examine the ways in which individual responses relate to wider social structures, if we are to fully understand both the opportunities and challenges which a focus on self health care poses for policies and for professionals.

Self-help

Self-help is perhaps the key concept with which to begin any discussion of developments in the field of self health care. It is a term which symbolizes the shift during the 1980s towards a much wider acceptance of a social model of health: a model which acknowledges and emphasizes that health and illness are not narrowly defined medical phenomenon, but are affected and influenced by social, economic, political and environmental factors (Beattie *et al.* 1992). Such a view is very much in keeping with the World Health Organization/UNICEF Declaration of Alma Ata on Primary Health Care, which made clear that health should be considered as 'a state of complete physical, mental and social well-being, and . . . a fundamental human right' (WHO 1978).

Self-help, then, concerns some of the ways and means by which one might be enabled to attain such a state of well-being. More particularly, it can be seen as one response to developments in health and social welfare that have tended to exclude and marginalize certain groups, older people included. It is also about affirming the abilities and capacities of individuals to continue helping themselves without inevitable recourse to formal health and welfare services. Self-help has also been conceptualized as a movement encompassing, as discussed further below, self-help groups, self-help organizations and alternative care.

Self-help groups

Here, we are concerned in effect with issues of scale and size when looking at the finer distinctions concerning groups, organizations and alternative forms of care. Purist self-help is, very literally, about helping oneself. However, the second half of the twentieth century witnessed a rapid growth in people coming together with a common aim or purpose into self-help groups of various kinds. This suggests that mutuality as opposed to simple self-interest has a part to play in both conceptual and developmental terms. Lock (1986) has noted that many definitions of self-help groups are long and intricate. One such comprehensive definition, quoted below in its entirety, is proposed by Katz and Bender (1976) who define them as:

> voluntary, small group structures for mutual aid and the accomplishment of a special purpose. They are usually formed by peers who have come together for mutual assistance in satisfying a common need, overcoming a common handicap or life-disrupting problem, and bringing about desired

social and/or personal change. The initiators and members of such groups perceive that their needs are not, or cannot be, met by or through existing social institutions. Self help groups emphasise face to face social interactions and the assumption of personal responsibility by members. They often provide material assistance, as well as emotional support; they are frequently 'cause-oriented', and promulgate an ideology or values through which members may attain an enhanced sense of personal identity.

(Katz and Bender 1976: 9)

Within the detail of this definition, Katz and Bender (1976) also crucially remind us that many self-help groups are initiated as a result of people feeling and recognizing that they are, in some way, powerless. Joining together in a group offers one means of beginning to challenge that perceived powerlessness. This point is made explicit by Butler and his colleagues (1979) who argue that self-help groups

typically arise as a spontaneous, grass-roots response to a specific need, and consist of persons who share mutual concerns . . . self help groups feature face-to-face interactions, emphasise personal participation, eschew bureaucratization, engage in selected actions, and often start up from a position of powerlessness.

(Butler *et al.* 1979: 100)

They also observe that while many self-help groups exist, only a few are designed specifically to meet the needs of older people. However, a great number are directed at helping chronically ill people and, as we have seen in Chapters 1 and 2, many sufferers of chronic conditions tend to be aged. Self-help groups thus have great potential for meeting some of the needs of this sector of the population.

North American work in the late 1970s can be contrasted with the somewhat simpler definitions of self-help which emerged in a British context in the following decade. Richardson and Goodman (1983), for example, contend that very complex definitions actually exclude many groups ordinarily seen as self-help. Linked with this, writers on both sides of the Atlantic were also concerned with delineating the characteristics of self-help groups. Knight and Hayes (1981) for example, outline seven key features:

1 They are voluntary.
2 Members have shared problems.
3 They have meetings for mutual benefit.
4 The helper/helped role is shared.
5 The group is concerned with constructive action towards shared goals.
6 Groups are self-run.
7 Groups exist without outside funding.

These characteristics, they argue, serve as a model against which actual groups can be compared, as in their own work on self-help community initiatives in four inner city areas of London, and their subsequent review of nine innovatory economic self-help projects (Knight and Hayes 1981, 1982).

Other researchers and writers on this topic have attempted to focus more precisely on self-help in relation to health. In the USA, in the latter half of the 1970s, Tracy and Gussow (1976) distinguished between two main types of what they called 'mutual help associations' providing services and support to patients and relatives: Type I were informal, loosely organized groups with small or non-existent budgets, and Type II were larger scale and with an emphasis on public education, fundraising, research, lobbying and legislative activities. This typology was subsequently expanded by Gartner and Reissman (1976), who subdivided Type I into four categories according to their particular orientations:

1 *Rehabilitative groups* – for conditions like strokes and mastectomy.
2 *Behaviour modification groups* – dealing with problems such as drugs, smoking, alcohol and eating conditions.
3 *Adjustment to lifestyle groups* – which would include, for example, women's groups and support groups for people who have been bereaved.
4 *Prevention and case finding* – which might include conditions such as hypertension.

A rather broader functional definition of what constitutes a self-help group is given by Vincent (1986) in her study of self-help groups in health care in the East Midlands of England. In this instance, she defines a 'prescriptive ideal' in which self-help groups are characterized along just three dimensions:

• Members share a problem.
• Reciprocity is the primary mode of exchange.
• Participative democracy informs organizational arrangements.

Groups are then defined as self-help if they have one or more of these features.

While defining terms is obviously important, and typologies can be more or less helpful, there are evident dangers in having either too broad or too narrow a definitional perspective. Too broad, and we potentially encompass almost any kind of group one might care to think about. Too narrow, and we risk excluding groups which may in fact espouse many of the features associated with self-help. Whatever definition or characteristics one adopts, it is also important to recognize that over time, such definitions may become outmoded by virtue of the fact that new forms of self-help activity are continually being developed (Posner 1989). Indeed, as far back as the mid-1970s Levy (1976) remarked that perhaps the most striking feature of self-help groups was their diversity – an observation which is no less true today. More recently, Gareth Williams (1989) has commented that self-help groups will tend to divide into those which focus very much on individual concerns, and those which are more directed at outside interests or dilemmas. Without wishing to split definitional hairs, it may be that outer directed groups such as these could more accurately be considered as coming within that part of the Hatch and Kickbusch (1983) self-help continuum which relates to self-help organizations.

Self-help organizations and pressure groups

Such groups and organizations obviously vary considerably in size and purpose. In relation to health, they may be organized around general or specific health care issues; they may focus on the organization of health care, on health promotion strategies, or on disease prevention. Often, they have an overt political purpose aimed at bringing about changes in the health care system and the larger society. In effect, this can be conceived as the action-oriented element of self-help, and is usually the most publicly visible element of the self-help continuum (Kickbusch and Hatch 1983). Perhaps the most developed examples of such organizations in Britain are those directed at supporting informal carers of various kinds. The Carers National Association, for example, takes a particular interest in the development and improvement of services to ease the burden on carers through things like increased respite care and support groups. It is also active in promoting training and information for professionals and carers, in producing guidelines for service providers and policy makers, and in campaigning for greater awareness of the needs of those whose interests they serve.

In the context of health, there are many self-help organizations and groups that one can point to. One observer claims that in Britain there are at least 1500 national self-help organizations, with over 25,000 regional branches (Lock 1986). The most visible tend to be those associated with women's health concerns, and have their basis in the women's health movement of the 1960s and 1970s. Issues about childbirth, contraception, abortion and maternity care were at the basis of the struggle in developed nations, to replace the medical view of women as inferior and sickly people, with a recognition of them as normal and healthy human beings. Doyal (1995) charts, in a global context, these women's movements for health. She shows that while much has been achieved – for example the National Women's Health Network in the USA now has 17,000 members and in Australia there is a National Women's Health Policy which emphasizes the creation and support of women's health centres – there is still continuing need for groups and organizations to press for fundamental changes to existing systems.

While in some ways it is possible to draw analogies between the women's health movement and what is happening today in respect of health and older people, historically, older people have been ill served by many of the groups and organizations purporting to serve their interests. In many instances, the public image of older people is of poor, lonely, disabled and unhealthy human beings, which suggests that we still have a long way to go in countering such negative attitudes. This is despite the developments in health promotion since the late 1980s charted in Chapter 2.

Alternative care

In considering the concept of alternative care, we need to distinguish between alternative services and alternative medicine. With regard to the former, many alternative care services have often been developed in the context of self-help groups and may, in fact, be directly provided by them. In essence, they constitute services which would otherwise not be available, or are services which promote other forms of treatment or care not provided by the formal health care system. An example of such a service is the development, in certain US states, of refuges for older people who are the victims of domestic violence.

In respect of alternative medicine, Pietroni (1995) has described its recent growth as, in part, an expression of patients or 'consumers' voting with their feet. In other words patients, because of their dissatisfaction with conventional medicine are, in effect 'pushed' to seek alternative ways of dealing with their condition. This runs counter to the widespread idea that users are somehow naïvely drawn or 'pulled' by the claims of alternative healers. Sharma's (1995) research confirms that many people who use such methods do so because of a variety of sources of dissatisfaction with orthodox medicine. In particular, conventional medicine's emphasis on cure as opposed to symptom relief may be inappropriate – especially for many older people suffering with chronic conditions such as arthritis. Alternative medicine takes a much more holistic approach to the health of the individual and offers a range of treatments based upon individual diagnosis as opposed to universal cure for particular ailments (Scrutton 1992).

Lay and volunteer care

Lay care is an overarching term, encompassing all the health care which we offer to each other either in everyday situations, or in more organized settings (Kickbusch and Hatch 1983). Research since the late 1970s has revealed the considerable extent to which older people in particular are reliant on such forms of care. In the early 1980s, it was estimated that between 60 and 90 per cent of all health care was provided by lay people (Levin and Idler 1981). Moreover, there is a growing body of research exploring what has been called the 'lay referral system' whereby people tend first to consult others in order to establish whether they are in fact 'ill' and, if so, what they might do about it (see, for example, Freidson 1970; Scambler *et al.* 1981; Sanders 1982). One such study reported that 71 per cent of the symptom episodes experienced by working class women, which eventually led to a consultation with a doctor, were first discussed with a lay person (Scambler *et al.* 1981). Similarly, the students in Sanders' (1982) study revealed that on average, they sought advice from three lay people about the symptoms they had suffered over the preceding year. They also reported receiving unsolicited medical advice from others and had, themselves, acted in this capacity (R.G.A. Williams 1983; Cornwell 1984).

Lay care not only consists of advice – whether consciously sought or unsolicited – but also includes actual support to other people and, in this sense, is sometimes regarded as synonymous with the concept of informal or nonprofessional care. Green's (1988) analysis of the 1985 General Household Survey originally drew professional and public attention to the 6 million people involved in such care of others. Before, but particularly since this publication, the debate has continued to rage around issues such as who exactly is involved in providing informal care; what they do or do not do; what the diversity of caring situations encompasses; how caring affects lay carers in psychological, emotional, physical, social and financial terms; and how policies and practice should respond to assist and support such 'voluntary' effort (Twigg 1998). Although there is not space here to consider these dimensions in detail it is evident that, however one attempts to 'cost' the value of informal or lay care, it saves the exchequer considerable sums of money. Indeed, some commentators have observed that without such lay and informal care, the health and welfare system would collapse (Qureshi and Walker 1989). Thus, we can conclude that lay care is in effect, the most substantive form of health and social care in most societies.

When lay care becomes somewhat more organized, we can recognize it as being forms of volunteer care provided by community members via the auspices of a particular group or agency. Examples here are numerous and might include church-based volunteers, voluntary agencies of various kinds, and people who offer their services to charities. In Britain, as in some other European countries, there is a long tradition of voluntary help and care-giving (Tinker 1992). In other cultural contexts, this may not be so marked although older people are often notable by their involvement in such voluntarism. In North America, for example, it is estimated that between one-third and two-fifths of older people volunteer through religious organizations, hospitals, schools and locally based programmes (Hooyman and Kiyak 1988; Herzog and House 1991). There are also some organizations composed entirely of older people. These include the Retired Senior Volunteer Programme (RSVP), which runs projects in nursing homes, schools, hospitals and day care facilities and supervises in excess of a quarter of a million volunteers, and the Senior Companion Program which provides peer help and assistance (Cox and Parsons 1994).

In Britain, the Carnegie Inquiry into the Third Age found that about four in ten people aged between 50 and 74 had volunteered in the previous year (Davis Smith 1992), and that older people spend much more time on their voluntary work than do younger adults (Lynn and Davis Smith 1991). Volunteers between the ages of 65 and 74 devote, on average, over five hours a week to this activity compared with an average for all other age groups of less than three hours. Moreover, the most popular areas for older volunteers to be involved in are the health and welfare fields, and in groups helping other elderly people (MORI 1990). The best known national and regional agencies in this field include organizations such as Age Concern, Help the Aged, Pensioners Link and the Beth Johnson Foundation, while there are also numerous other local groups around the UK. While many of these kinds of voluntary activities involve health, it is the specific development of self-care and self health care activities which provides the most acutely health focused element of the self-help continuum.

Self-care and self health care

Self-care and self health care are the central concepts with which the bulk of this book is concerned. As noted earlier, there is now a growing body of literature in Europe and North America addressing the theory, methodology and practice of self-care on which we can usefully draw. In 1989, for example, a special issue of the journal *Social Science and Medicine* appeared. In this issue, Kickbusch (1989) provided an interesting historical overview of the development of self-care, tracing the parallels between it and the academic discovery of poverty in the 1960s. She argued that, like poverty, self-care has always been with us but that it was not until the late 1970s that the self-help and women's health movements brought it to the attention of a wider public. At this time though, only a few programmes were designed specifically with older people in mind, and these were almost exclusively confined to North America (Butler *et al.* 1979). Savo (1985) has argued that the early development of these programmes can be viewed along a spectrum from professionally controlled, clinically oriented approaches focusing on personal health behaviour at one end, to community development programmes at the other. In Britain too, it is possible to trace the strong influence of community development work from the 1960s onwards, again emerging initially as a response to poverty and urban deprivation (Hart and Bond 1995). However, as with any 'new' discovery, definitional sophistication and research approaches take some time to develop.

Self-care

In the 1970s and early 1980s, self-care tended to be defined very much in individual terms. Levin *et al.* (1976, cited in Holstein 1986: 49) described it thus: 'as a process whereby a lay person functions on his/her own behalf in health promotion and prevention and in disease detection and treatment at the level of the primary health resource in the health care system'. Other writers argued similarly that self-care should be seen as 'the individual health behaviour component of self help' (Dean 1983: 20); and that it 'may be viewed in terms of the individual defining, planning, and being responsible for a range of health behaviours' (Phillipson 1984: 1).

However, defining self-care simply in terms of what people can do for themselves was quickly seen to be inadequate. To do so can, by association, easily become victim-blaming as well as providing a rationale for further cutting of health and welfare services. Thus, the notion of purist self-care became supplemented by considering ways in which the individual interacted with others. In order to distinguish it from self-help, emphasis was laid on the informal and unorganized nature of self-care:

> Self-care refers to unorganized health activities and health-related decision-making by individuals, families, neighbours, friends, colleagues at work, etc.; it encompasses self-medication, self-treatment, social support in illness, first aid in a 'natural setting', i.e. the normal social context of people's everyday lives.
>
> (Kickbusch and Hatch 1983: 4)

By the mid-1980s, Illsley (1986) was boldly claiming that 'the meaning of self-care is clear' and defined it as being 'concentrated upon the individual and upon the individual's knowledge, motivation and actions to nurture body and mind by preventive behaviour and by treatment, autonomously, but in cooperation with others'.

However, others who contributed to the volume from which this quotation is taken also made attempts to modify the definition further (Dean *et al.* 1986). Self-care was defined by some to include what one does for family and friends (Katz 1986), as well as decisions regarding seeking professional care, and partnerships between the individual and professionals (Dean 1986, 1989). Dean's work also drew attention to the importance of self-care including decisions on the part of individuals to do nothing:

> Self-care involves the range of activities individuals undertake to enhance health, prevent disease, evaluate symptoms and restore health. These activities are undertaken by lay people on their own behalf, either separately or in participation with professionals. Self-care includes decisions to do nothing, self-determined actions to promote health or treat illness, and decisions to seek advice in lay, professional and alternative care networks, as well as evaluation of and decisions regarding action based on that advice.
>
> (Dean 1986: 82)

While what one does for family and friends may more appropriately be considered in the lay care part of the self-help continuum, it is evident that issues concerning the boundaries of definitions are important if we are not to be left with rather more conceptual confusion than definitional clarity. Highlighting the link with professional care and with other individuals is important in drawing attention to the wider social and political contexts within which self-care activities are pursued. It emphasizes the fact that self-care is active social behaviour, and behaviour which does not take place in a political and societal vacuum (Kickbusch 1989). Yet, despite increasing definitional sophistication in the literature, it is still the case that 'while many authors have attempted to define self-care, no broadly accepted definition has been developed' (Mockenhaupt 1993: 5).

One way forward is to consider more precisely what it is we undertake when we engage in self-care. However, just to confuse matters still further, it has also been observed that self-care itself can equally be applied to health or medicine. In the 1990s, we therefore had two subdivisions of self-care ('medical self-care' and 'health self-care') to consider (Vickery and Levinson 1993).

Medical self-care

Defined as being 'what people do to recognize, prevent, treat, and manage their own health problems' (Mettler and Kemper 1993: 7), medical self-care includes a number of identifiable components. Vickery and Levinson (1993) detail five elements, which are discussed below:

1 *Self-management* – the ability to manage part or all of a medical problem on one's own. This involves assessing its nature and severity and/or treating it.
2 *Informed choice* – so that the individual can make a decision based on full knowledge of the probable benefits and risks of each option.
3 *Self-efficacy* – believing that one can effectively deal with a particular health problem or situation.
4 *Screening* – detection of hidden disease by testing apparently healthy people.
5 *Provider information* – the collation of facts which might be useful in choosing a health professional.

Although, on the face of it, *self-management* might appear a relatively simple undertaking, it effectively means both learning about and practising certain skills. It also involves caring for one's condition (for example, by taking medication, exercising or observing a particular diet), while also maintaining one's normal lifestyle and dealing with the emotions which learning to live with a particular condition or disease might generate (Corbin and Strauss 1988). Self-management, therefore, goes beyond just learning about the condition and, to be successful, it requires change from both the individual and the health professionals (Lorig 1993). There are also a number of limitations to self-management which it is important to mention here. These include practical considerations such as whether equipment is available and, if so, whether the individual has the skills to use it, together with legal and ethical limitations involving the sharing of medical knowledge and questions of medical liability.

The concept of *informed choice* is one which has to be considered within the context of differing cultural, value and belief systems. However, it is evident that where individuals do have choices, medical personnel sometimes treat this kind of information as their exclusive property. From Britain, for example, there is evidence that doctors do not give older patients as much information as they need or want, and that their opinions are not taken seriously (Wenger 1988; Sidell 1991). Older women in particular are especially dependent on their doctors, and often feel disappointed and dissatisfied with the treatment they receive (Sidell 1993). The same point applies to the health needs and differing cultural concepts of health and disease held by minority ethnic older people.

Many of the ways in which we respond to professionals have to do with the extent to which we believe we can effectively deal with a health problem ourselves. At bottom, *self-efficacy* is about one's level of self-confidence, and enhancing self-confidence is a goal at the heart of many self-help activities. Since the 1980s, we have seen a veritable explosion of self-help manuals purporting to help people reawaken their dormant abilities and become more effective at overseeing their own health. While older people have not generally been the focus of much of this literature, they are now being more overtly targeted (see, for example, Fries 1989; Phillips and Rakusen 1989; Shapiro 1989). Like self-management though, self-efficacy alone is insufficient. It has to be an integral part of a wider programme which also looks at social and environmental approaches.

Among such approaches, the issues around *screening* can be seen to feature prominently in recent literature relating to health – and particularly the health of older women. The basic rationale for screening hinges on the fact that many diseases are best treated as early as possible. A wide variety of screening is now available and individuals exercise their option to self-care when they decide whether or not to go. However, a great deal of research questions the value of screening procedures, and reveals the ways in which older people are discriminated against in screening campaigns. For example, while the United States, the Netherlands and Sweden routinely screen women over the age of 65 for breast cancer, this is not the case in Britain (Sidell 1995). Some people also distinguish between a case-finding as opposed to screening approach, given the fact that there are marked differences in individual risk factors.

Finally, in Vickery and Levinson's (1993) formulation, much of medical self-care is essentially about trying to ensure that we have adequate *information* to help us choose and receive the best quality of professional health care available. In reality though, one rarely sees health providers often enough in order to be able to make a judgement about their capabilities. Quality is therefore a very difficult issue for the individual to assess fully.

Health self-care

Health self-care, by contrast, concerns first and foremost the behavioural and lifestyle choices we make which in turn affect our health (Vickery and Levinson 1993). These are influenced by a complex interplay of socio-demographic, cultural, social, environmental and political forces. More than this, though, health self-care concerns the decisions that individuals make about the extent to which they will or will not become involved in trying to change the wider environmental, social and structural inequalities which impinge on health. It means 'deciding whether and how to participate in an appropriate political process to correct the condition' (Vickery and Levinson 1993: 54). This places health self-care firmly within the wider arena of health promotion, but in a view of health promotion which, as we have seen in Chapter 2, embraces a structural analysis and goes beyond the notion of individual responsibility for health. It also leads us into a consideration of how, and in what ways, self health care either echoes or is distinguishable from self-care.

Self health care

A working definition of self health care is given in the World Health Organization's manual compiled by Coppard *et al.* (1984: 3). They consider it as: 'all the actions and decisions that an individual takes to prevent, diagnose, and treat personal ill health; all individual behaviours calculated to maintain and improve health; and decisions to access and use both informal support systems and formal medical services'.

This immediately resonates with the definition of medical self-care above, and Coppard *et al.* (1984) go on to delineate what might usefully be included under the remit of self health care skills. They suggest that there is a measure of general agreement on this issue, and that self health care involves five quite specific individual skills:

1 *Simple diagnostic skills* – which the individual can practise in making an estimate of his/her health status, such as checking temperature and pulse rate, breast self-examination.
2 *Skills relevant to simple acute conditions* – for example treatment of the common cold and everyday illnesses, first aid for non-life-threatening injuries.
3 *Skills needed to treat chronic illnesses* – such as self-monitoring, following prescribed regimens.
4 *Skills required for disease prevention and health promotion* – for example exercise,

diet, avoiding tobacco and alcohol abuse, good dental hygiene, healthy life-styles.

5 *Health information skills* – such as knowledge about what steps to take prior to seeking professional treatment, how to obtain health information, how to gain access to formal care.

The means to impart, and then to reinforce and develop such skills, are poten-tially endless. They could include educational initiatives, health behaviour modification programmes, the use of self-care manuals and books, health courses, resource centres for health, involvement in volunteer groups, peer counselling, self-management of conditions ranging from stress to arthritis, and social and leisure activities. However, despite the growing number of developments across Europe, North America and Australasia (Hickey 1993), British work in these areas is still very limited.

What is clearly evident though is that such skills development cannot take place within a social vacuum. Consequently, self health care can be seen very much as an integral part of the more general practice of lay care outlined above, and of the wider concept of health promotion. This implies that the individual, while taking responsibility for his or her own health, also shares it with others. The logical extension of this is that rather than being outside the remit of health and social care professionals, the encouragement of such skills among older people could and should be facilitated by a variety of staff.

Taken together, self-care and self health care can be seen to offer a challenge to the dominance of the biomedical model. Engagement in such activities chal-lenges authority and professional knowledge. However, it is also aimed, in the words of Lorig (1993: 13), 'at helping the participant become an active, not adversarial, partner with healthcare providers'. In this respect, it is a mistake to see self-care and self health care as a means of replacing professional care (Bernard and Phillipson 1991). Rather, it can be seen both as an integral element in the arguments put forward by critical gerontologists which suggest that people can exert more control over their lives in old age through a combi-nation of self-care, statutory support and political empowerment (Phillipson and Strang 1986); and as an important dimension of a new public health per-spective which seeks to reassert the influence of social and environmental factors on health (Ashton and Seymour 1988; Kickbusch 1989).

The nature and limitations of existing research

The definitional developments discussed above have not taken place in iso-lation, either from practical developments or from research. Broadly speaking, it is possible to critique the present state of research on self health care accord-ing to two main dimensions: the kinds of research undertaken, and the methods used. While some readers might perhaps think it churlish to highlight gaps or deficiencies in the research and developments to date, it is important not to fall into the trap of self-complacency, particularly when many develop-ments are poorly evaluated if at all (Bernard and Phillipson 1991). Moreover, it is incumbent upon us all, whether practitioners or researchers, to reflect criti-cally on what is still poorly articulated and understood in research terms, as well as on what projects and programmes have undoubtedly achieved.

The nature of research

Historically, the nature of much research on self health care has been oriented towards descriptive (some would even say anecdotal) accounts of developments and practices. Within this, though, there are discernible foci through which research in this area has passed. In particular, this has included concerns with illness and with health-related behaviours; with individual risk factors; with interventions; with preventive and health-promoting approaches; and with work in particular settings. To a certain extent, this body of research reflects the explosion of practical interest in the topic, with a great deal of work being done since the 1980s around self health care projects and models, and on the publication of 'how to' manuals. Some of these projects are detailed in Chapter 4 but, although there are now many interesting and innovative programmes, it is probably still the case that this is an 'under-researched and under-evaluated' area (Glendenning 1985: 7).

In the early days, research tended to be concerned primarily with illness and with health-related behaviour on the part of individuals. Set against a background of rising health care expenditure, a key concern was to highlight the use older people made of health services: research on utilization was paramount. Alongside this, there was also a focus on single problems faced by older people, e.g. arthritis, as opposed to more generalized health difficulties. Through patient education, the emphasis was on getting people to change particular unhealthy practices, instead of addressing problems in their wider personal and societal contexts.

Arising out of this historical basis, it is evident that a limitation of much early research was the emphasis it placed on the role of the individual. Consideration of wider socio-economic and structural factors was notable by its absence: findings concentrated on what the individual needed to do in order to improve his or her own health status, make more efficient use of resources, and so on. The links between individual behaviour and the broader social and environmental contexts in which we live out our lives were, for the most part, overlooked. Similarly, individual solutions as opposed to structural interventions, were usually the major recommendations. As such, research findings often served to reinforce the victim-blaming which still, some would argue, strongly tinges policies.

Related to this, the terms within which early research was conceived, meant that self health care was often looked at only in respect of how people responded to symptoms of illness. It was also regarded as almost the direct opposite of professional help (Dean 1992). More recent research has broadened to include examinations of how people respond to everyday symptoms, and to considerations of the various practices adopted to deal with these symptoms, particularly self-medication (Edwardson 1993). However, as has already been noted, self-medication is only one of a possible range of self-treatments. Dietary responses, use of alternative treatments and complementary therapies, home remedies and the avoidance of harmful practices, all are areas worthy of more extensive study (Dean 1992). Although research to date indicates that the majority of such responses are safe and appropriate, we also need to know more about the outcomes of these self-treatments. Specifically,

Hickey (1993) contends that we need more convincing data about therapeutic outcomes, as well as how such treatments might affect the incidence and progression of chronic disease and functional capacities. Alongside this, research on the cost effectiveness or otherwise of self-care responses and treatments is still in its infancy.

A further area of research (as yet underdeveloped) concerns the impact of cohort differences. People who are old today have grown up in a social and political climate which, in Britain at least, means that they share certain experiences: two world wars and the emergence of the welfare state in particular (Sidell 1995). While it is ultimately unhelpful to consider all older people as a group with consistent beliefs and views about health and illness, it is important to try to tease out some of the patterns and common influences. There is evidence, for example, that many older people internalize the ageist assumptions of society which links chronological age with inevitable decline and disability. Negative stereotypes of ageing, and negative approaches to growing older, may influence responses to health education and health promotion. Older people will, for example, be less likely to engage in such activities if they believe that their future expectations are restricted in various ways (Rakowski and Hickey 1980). Sidell (1995: 32) also observes that today's older people are 'under great pressure to cope stoically with ill-health, not to complain and to suffer in silence. They are also under great pressure not to make too many demands upon the health and welfare services and become a burden to the rest of society'.

These beliefs, pressures and expectations may well be very different for people who are currently only approaching later life (Evandrou 1997). We therefore need much greater consideration than we have had up till now, about the ways in which being a member of a particular cohort might influence our approach to both health and illness, and our propensity to engage in and with self health care practices.

Research methods

Not surprisingly, given the above discussion, research methods too have undergone something of a transformation since the late 1970s. Put simplistically, much of the early research tended to be extremely quantitative in nature and concerned with what could be 'objectively' measured. Epidemiological methods, for example, tell us convincingly about the prevalence of disabilities, and about the relationships between morbidity, mortality and risk factors. Experimental and intervention studies, meanwhile, have demonstrated that things like low intensity exercise are of benefit to the health status of older people. Yet, even with increasing technological sophistication, with our ability to computer model how people might respond to and deal with a whole gamut of illness symptoms, and with the advent of extremely large-scale and cross-national studies, we are still some way from being able to appreciate fully the essentially subjective nature of self health care in the lives of older people. This suggests that quantitative methods need to be complemented by qualitative investigations which seek to address issues such as the meanings ascribed by older people to a range of self health care practices, and the ways in which personal biographies, health beliefs and personal situations influence self health care responses (Biggs *et al.* 1998).

Latterly too, practical developments themselves have become more wide-ranging and comprehensive. While this provides a more accurate reflection of the place of health and illness in people's lives, it poses considerable dilemmas for research methodology. In effect, it becomes more and more difficult to isolate elements for research scrutiny, and ways and means need to be found to conceptualize and examine some of the more sophisticated and multivariate dimensions now encompassed by the self health care movement.

The final point of this brief overview concerns the shift during the period since the appearance of the seminal volume on self-care (Dean *et al.* 1986) in research focus. While it is evident that we have moved, for the most part, beyond simple descriptive research and away from an emphasis on single problems, patient education and health care utilization, researchers are still left with particular challenges. In the conclusion to his preface in the self health care volume, Illsley (1986) noted that 'what is now needed . . . is evaluation' – an observation which remains just as pertinent today, when we consider the paucity of research associated with many of the self health care programmes operating around the world. In the 1990s too, the concept of 'empowerment' has entered our vocabulary. This notion has been conceptualized and operationalized in various ways through, for example, ideas about patient autonomy, consumer rights and user participation. However, with regard to self health care, the concept of empowerment is poorly articulated or understood. Nor, it has to be conceded, has it been looked at empirically. Both programme evaluation, and empowerment as a focus for such research, are issues taken up again in the second half of this book. Before doing so, however, this chapter concludes with a brief résumé of why what I term 'self empowered health behaviour' may be an appropriate way forward for both research and developments in this field (Bernard 1988).

Conclusion: self-empowered health behaviour – one way forward?

Having reviewed the health of older people in both this and the preceding two chapters, there is now an urgent need to move forward both conceptually and empirically. From our considerations in Chapter 1 of the health experiences of older people, we can conclude that:

- Ageing is not inevitably associated with negative expectations of physical and mental decline, disease and disability.
- Staying healthy is of prime importance to older people.
- There is great variation in the manner, extent and timing of how age-related changes affect the lives of older people.
- Older people, like younger people, conceptualize health in very broad terms, encompassing social, emotional and spiritual dimensions as well as biological and physiological.

In Chapter 2, we discussed two major aspects of health: developments in health policy and developments in health promotion. From this review, it was evident that, on the one hand, older people have become increasingly disenchanted with aspects of conventional medicine while on the other, health promotion is beginning to be seen as a worthwhile activity. The concept of 'empowerment', to which we have again returned at the end of this chapter, was offered as a key concept to link these various dimensions together. Again, it is possible to summarize a number of points arising out of this discussion:

- Health promotion is an umbrella concept encompassing individual, social, economic and environmental aspects of health.
- Health promotion consists of a number of related activities and components and has four strands: health protection, prevention, education and preservation.
- Older people have largely been excluded from the arena of health promotion.
- Although older people, like most people, take care of their own health for most of the time, they are also the biggest per capita users of conventional health care resources.
- Empowerment is central to thinking about the ways in which older people might be supported in their use of both formal and informal health care services, for the benefit of themselves and others.

This chapter has extended the review of health among older people to a consideration of perspectives on self-help and self health care. The self-help continuum, like health promotion itself, encompasses a range of behaviours and activities from the individual level up to and including various forms of community and wider societal action. The women's health movement is perhaps the clearest example of the self-help continuum in operation. In addition, the growing interest in self health care reflects gradual changes in attitude towards ageing and old age, with a questioning by both older people and their carers of some of the traditional stereotypes. As with health promotion, self health care cannot be divorced from the wider societal, political and environmental contexts within which it has to operate.

Thus, what stands out from this examination of the dimensions of health and of self health care are a number of key issues. Drawing them together, we can see that in essence, the ability of people to engage in self health care depends on them being able to do the following:

- *Gain access* – to personal and community resources and networks; to physical resources; to information; to people; and to one's own wishes and feelings.
- *Get support* – both practically and emotionally to fix and translate desired goals into behaviour and actions.
- *Obtain information* – about self; others; available support and community resources.
- *Make choices* – from among various options.
- *Develop skills* – to enable one to choose and maintain optimum health; practical, personal, interpersonal and situational skills.
- *Participate* – in whatever way, and to whatever extent, one desires.
- *Achieve empowerment* – through raised awareness, knowledge, understanding and competence.

In conclusion, it is therefore suggested that these seven dimensions should underpin attempts to develop more dynamic models, policies and practices aimed at enhancing the health and well-being of people as they age. This 'self-empowered health behaviour' approach builds on earlier work around life skills development (Hopson and Scally 1981) and health skills (Anderson 1986), in an attempt to bridge the gap between private and public action in the health arena, and between notions of individual responsibility for health and underlying structural and political dimensions. It reasserts the importance of considering the individual within the context of his or her own social nexus, helping us to examine ways in which self health care develops over time and how it contributes to the construction of meaning and self-identity (Dill *et al.* 1995). For those of us interested in self-care and self health care, it therefore implies that we have to try and engage in the difficult juggling act of attending to both personal experiences of health alongside a structural analysis. In this sense, 'self-care can be promoted as a pathway to empowerment' (Mettler and Kemper 1993: 10) while also being seen as empowering in and of itself: 'as an important addition to human competence and skills' (Kickbusch 1989: 129). Finally, such an approach potentially lends itself to being translated into criteria against which to assess the impact of any new project: criteria which form the framework for the monitoring and evaluation of the Self Health Care in Old Age Project detailed in the second half of this book.

4

Developments in self health care

Introduction

We have seen in Chapter 3 that the notion of self health care has undergone a certain amount of modification and refinement since the late 1970s. Emerging from the broader concept of self-help, and viewed as an integral element of health promotion and the new public health, the role of self health care in the lives of older people has become ever more visible. However, conceptual and research developments cannot and do not occur in isolation from practice. Over the years, the concerns and issues identified in previous chapters have found expression in a number of comprehensive programmes. It is therefore the aim of this chapter to present some brief case studies. These programmes and projects illustrate the diversity of activity and research which now goes under the umbrella of self health care, as well as providing the context for the Beth Johnson Foundation's own Self Health Care in Old Age Project.

As is abundantly clear, many of the developments in self health care have come from North America. From among the myriad of projects across this vast continent, this chapter describes three long-standing developments (two from the United States and one from Canada). For readers wishing to learn more there is literature, including directories and annotated bibliographies, which gives details of programmes across North America (see, for example, National Institute on Aging 1984; Savo 1984). Also described is one of the formative developments from Britain in the 1980s, and a more recent project from Israel begun in the early 1990s.

The selection of these projects is in no sense random. On the contrary, they are a very personal choice. They have been chosen essentially because I have, since the mid-1980s, spoken to, and corresponded with, a number of the key personnel involved with the research and development of these projects.

Readers will not find examples of European projects here, but may refer to publications from Age Concern and EurolinkAge and to Kickbusch and Hatch (1983). Accounts of some self-help and health-related projects from other parts of the world will be found in Tout (1993).

Starting where people are: the Yale Self Care Education Project (United States)

Like a number of the initiatives in the United States in the late 1970s, the Yale Self Care Education Project was a response to what had become known as the Health Activation Program for adults. This was initially developed in 1970 by a medical practitioner, Keith Sehnert, and was based on his book entitled *How To Be Your Own Doctor (Sometimes)* (Sehnert and Eisenberg 1975). The programme was widely adopted by health educators across the United States and received a great deal of publicity. By 1982, it was estimated that 2500 such programmes were in existence (Levin 1982). The 32-hour, 16-session course aimed to help adults:

- accept more individual responsibility for their own health care and that of their family;
- learn skills in observation and description, together with the handling of common illnesses, injuries and emergencies;
- apply basic medical knowledge about common health problems;
- develop the more economical and effective use of health care resources, services and medications.

(Nocerino *et al.* 1977)

The development of such a course – or the Sehnert model as it became known – needs to be seen within the historical and policy context of the time. It was based very much on a traditional didactic model of health education with an emphasis, as we saw earlier, on altering individual health behaviours. This is a top-down model, a model that tries to anticipate individual needs and interests, and then leads to a professionally constructed and delivered programme of education. While such a model has the advantage of being easily replicable in other locations, the Health Activation Program failed to address the maintenance of health in a wider sense, and empowerment was incidental rather than central to the process of education (Levin 1982). The programme was also criticized for its white middle-class orientation, for its limited conceptualization of what constitutes health and self health care skills, and for its failure to have any impact on the social and community structures which affect the health of individuals.

By contrast, the Yale Project begins from the premise that empowerment (or self-empowered health behaviour) can come about only if people have control over 'the content, methods and outcome criteria' (Levin 1982: 4) of self-care education programmes. Lowell Levin, then Professor of Public Health in the Department of Epidemiology and Public Health at Yale University, persuaded the W K Kellogg Foundation to fund a three-year demonstration project at four different health facilities. The overriding aim of the project was 'the establishment of a model of self-care education which was truly empowering and firmly fixed in the social centre of the community, its values, its style of problem-solving, and its diverse subpopulations' (Levin 1982: 4). Underlying this were a number of more specific objectives:

- To test how valid the assumptions are that interest in self-care cuts across sociocultural lines, and that health empowerment develops from a client-centred approach to health education.
- To learn how to develop such programmes particularly in relation to strategies of client recruitment, encouragement of client control, the identification and support of client preferred methodologies, and client defined criteria for measuring outcomes.
- To examine the impact of this approach on the community, and on the sponsoring facility.

Four different sites were selected as the locations for the project, although each was operationally linked to a central administrative unit in the university and to Lowell Levin, the principal investigator. Briefly the four sites were as follows:

- *Fair Haven Community Health Clinic* – a 'free clinic' established in 1971 by a group of residents, serving a poor working-class, inner-city community where no health services existed. The population of 28,000 was ethnically mixed, with 20 per cent black, 40 per cent Spanish speaking, 40 per cent white Italians and a substantial proportion of people over the age of 65. It also operated a satellite clinic serving 2300 elderly people in Bella Vista, 'the largest high-rise housing complex in New England' (Savo 1984: 39).
- *Hill Health Centre* – opened in 1968 and serving a poor working-class population, many of whom were reliant on welfare. The population of 21,000 consisted of approximately 49 per cent black, 12 per cent white, 36 per cent Spanish speaking and 4 per cent 'other'.
- *Griffin Hospital* – a 254-bed general hospital serving a population of 80,000 in the old industrial area of the Lower Naugatuck Valley. Five communities, approximately 10–15 miles from the city of New Haven, make up the population which is ethnically mixed, and with moderate to low incomes.
- *Yale Health Plan* – a facility provided by the university for its 25,000 students, faculty members, staff and their families. This largely middle-class group was provided with health education and hospital services.

Each site was overseen by a site director, and was responsible for developing its own programmes in response to the diverse needs of the local communities. As an illustration, a total of 139 distinct activities were undertaken by the four sites from June 1981 to the end of May 1982.

Developments at Bella Vista serve as a case study of the importance of beginning with the needs and wishes of older people themselves (Savo 1983, 1984, 1985). Prior to the arrival of Cynthia Savo as part-time self-care coordinator, the residents of the complex (75 per cent of whom were women) had been offered certain health education activities by the nurses and nutritionists associated with the clinic. These included an exercise programme, a weight loss group, and sessions on specific diseases such as arthritis and diabetes. Given the large numbers of people in this complex, the response rate was very poor. Savo's initial task therefore was not to put on further activities but to begin by finding out what the residents themselves wanted.

From among the residents, 70 people were selected for interview. They had been identified as 'natural helpers' and were people to whom others turned for information, advice, support and leadership. They included people such as volunteer receptionists at the clinic and resident security guards. Through the interviews Savo, and the students who were working with her, learnt that many of the residents suffered a great deal of stress when moving to the scheme. These stresses were often the result of various losses: of one's home, possessions, spouse, and pets. Consequently, a stress-management group was established which evolved into a weekly drop-in discussion group. The group incorporated relaxation techniques, massage and problem-solving sessions, together with invited speakers on special topics. With an advisory group of 12 residents, other activities were also initiated in the complex including a cardiopulmonary resuscitation (CPR) programme, teaching of the Heimlich manoeuvre to be able to deal with anyone choking should the need arise, sessions on women's health, and an ethnic recipe contest.

In order to examine the aims and objectives of the Yale Project, a broad evaluation strategy was drawn up (Levin 1982). Both quantitative and qualitative measures were used, with the intention of demonstrating the process of development of the project over time. It was felt to be fundamentally important that the evaluation should not be too intrusive or undermine those involved with the project. Regular feedback was built into the research strategy, and data collection tools underwent continual modification in response to the needs of staff and participants. Data collection techniques, coding procedures and the interpretation of data were adapted over time, as the nature of the activities themselves changed and developed. The findings from the evaluation inform us about the following:

- *Programme development* – how people became aware of what was available; why they did or did not take part; what the activities consisted of; participants' views of the activities; and how the projects related to, and networked with, their local communities.
- *Participant characteristics* – socio-demographic data concerning numbers; ages; sex; ethnic group; social class; locational context.
- *Interest in self-care education* – nature of activities at each site (personal and family health – self-care skills, nutrition, weight control, first aid; specific concerns – self-help groups, stress management; fitness – dance, exercise, yoga; and leadership – training trainers, involvement in advisory groups); educational methods used and preferred (such as lectures, discussions, experiential learning, mutual support).
- *Changes in individual empowerment* – definitions of health; use of information learnt and skills acquired; sharing of information and skills with others; utilization of health services; interaction with health professionals.
- *Changes in group empowerment* – nature of the groups; involvement of participants as teachers or helpers; continued involvement with the project; extension of group activities on an ad hoc basis.

By so doing, this project clearly demonstrated the wide social appeal which self-care has, and the ways in which it can be developed with groups who have not traditionally been involved with health education initiatives. It also reveals the fact that health issues and concerns cannot be divorced from other aspects of community life. As Levin (1982) concludes in the final report on the programme:

> Our clients became our teachers. The 'curricula' that emerged were theirs and educational methods followed their preferences . . . Our clients have helped us redefine health promotion by showing us that health care practices and health promoting behaviours are part of the same reality in daily living.
>
> (Levin 1982: 42)

Listening and empowering: the Tenderloin Senior Organizing Project (United States)

The second US project is another well-documented development in this field, the Tenderloin Senior Organizing Project (TSOP). It was initiated in 1979 by Professor Meredith Minkler and her students, and operated formally up until 1996. The overview given here is drawn from her address to the British Society of Gerontology's annual conference in 1995, from some of the articles that have appeared since the project's inception (Savo 1984; Minkler 1985, 1992, 1995, 1996) and from personal correspondence.

The Tenderloin is a district of San Francisco, a 45-block area which for decades has suffered from a shifting low income population of homeless people, ex-offenders, prostitutes, drug addicts, former mental patients and Indo-Chinese refugees. Among its many problems, the district was notable for its high levels of crime. It is also home to approximately 8000 elderly men and women who, for the most part, live in what are termed 'single room occupancy' (SRO) hotels. In other words, they inhabit what are often extremely run down rooms, many of which lack private kitchen or bathroom facilities. In contrast with most communities of older people, the Tenderloin has an excess of men compared with women. Many of them retired from the navy, settling in San Francisco because it was their favourite port. These elderly residents faced considerable problems: high rates of alcoholism, depression and other illnesses, together with extreme social isolation, poor nutrition, transport problems, difficulties in obtaining medical care and, above all, fear of crime.

With her students at the Berkeley School of Public Health, University of California, Meredith Minkler began a project designed to address the inter-related problems of poor health, social isolation and powerlessness. The project was conceived as a practical application of Freire's (1973) philosophy of 'education for critical consciousness'. Although this has remained as the key theoretical orientation of the project, it has proved to have limitations as well as advantages when applied to work of this nature (Minkler 1985). There were three main goals of the project:

• To improve the physical, mental and emotional health of residents, by increasing social support and providing relevant health education.

- To facilitate individual and community empowerment by helping residents to identify common problems or needs, and to collectively seek solutions to them.
- To provide a model of university/community cooperation through which this project could be replicated, to the advantage of both student volunteers and low income elderly people in their communities.

The project began with students offering to hold informal coffee hours or discussion groups in the hotel lobbies, once a week. Working within a community development tradition, it was essential that students establish high levels of trust between themselves and the residents before being able to effectively help them to examine in detail the problems they faced. After about a year of informal interaction, the residents formed themselves into a club which held regular discussions, showed films and organized parties. As levels of trust increased, residents began to share their personal concerns much more, and the students were able to ask about the major health problems which they faced. Much to their surprise, the overwhelming response to this question was 'crime'. Even when the students politely reworded their enquiry and said, 'You misunderstood, we were asking about health problems', the residents were adamant that crime was their biggest health problem (Minkler 1996: 475). It meant that they could not go out of doors without being mugged, and were consequently unable to get to a doctor, go for a walk or even get an evening meal (Minkler 1995).

Had the students and staff failed to hear what was being said to them, the project would probably have foundered at this point. Instead, residents were helped to organize a community meeting on the subject of crime which received a great deal of coverage in the media. Fifty residents attended and, from the meeting, they developed a list of recommendations. They also organized themselves into a formal coalition across different hotels which they named 'Tenderloin Tenants for Safer Streets'. Members met with the mayor and the chief of police and, as an immediate result, there was an increase in foot patrol officers and the police agreed to make regular visits to the hotels in order to get to know the residents.

Towards the end of 1982, the residents began the 'Safehouse Project', recruiting a range of places where people could seek refuge if they were, for example, being followed. Over 50 local shops and agencies agreed to be part of this project, including local stores, churches, bars, restaurants and other community facilities. Safehouses were identified by a sign in the window, which informed people that an emergency telephone call could be made from inside. These initiatives around crime prevention were credited with much of the 18 per cent drop in the crime rate in this area during the first twelve months of their operation.

Although a grassroots, university-sponsored health education project, TSOP evolved to become a formally constituted voluntary organization after some five years of operation. Reasons for this included the need to have a full-time paid coordinator for an ever-growing initiative; money to expand the training of volunteers (by 1985, more than 200 students studying public health and related subjects had worked with the project for between three months and two years), and to engage in evaluative research and further activities. By formalizing the organization in this way, it was also feasible to engage in longer-term planning, fundraising and more extensive publicity. Thus, by the mid-1980s it was possible to identify four distinct phases through which the project had passed, phases which illustrate the necessity of working in a detailed and sensitive way if real longer-term benefits are to be reaped.

- *Phase 1: Gaining entree and legitimacy* – doing detailed groundwork and working through, and with, established and respected agencies and/or individuals.
- *Phase 2: Initial community development* – work in individual hotels by means of informal interaction, in order to get to know residents and establish trust.
- *Phase 3: Inter-hotel coalition building and social action* – facilitation of a community-wide forum on crime which achieved both short and long-term results, and led to the creation of the Safehouse Project.
- *Phase 4: Private incorporation as a community-based organization* – formalizing the activities of the project into an organization with a full-time paid coordinator and resources for training, evaluation and further action.

During the last decade of its existence, TSOP not only consolidated its early developments but also considerably expanded its activities. As time went on, residents became less dependent on outside facilitators and greatly expanded their activities into other health-related projects. This included a focus on nutrition with weekly mini-markets being run in hotel lobbies so that residents could buy fresh fruit and vegetables; the establishment of a cooperative breakfast programme which qualified them for participation in a food bank; and the collation and subsequent publication of a 'no-cook' cookbook. A health promotion resource centre was set up and residents successfully campaigned for improved bus services, for hot water to be turned on in a building which had been without it for ten years, and for compensation for a lift which had been out-of-service for five months. Minkler (1996: 476) also notes that, in its latter years, residents organized themselves to protest against unfair increases in rent, and won an out-of-court settlement against a prestigious local law school which owned housing for older people in the district, but had reneged on its promise about security.

TSOP illustrates most graphically the way in which self health care cannot be divorced from a wider consideration of structural factors. There are very real limits to the amount of individual responsibility that residents in the Tenderloin district were and are able to take, to maintain and improve their health. Their living conditions, and features of their wider environment – particularly the high crime rates and poor access to services – mean that their abilities were severely constrained. Yet, even within these limits, the elderly residents of this district continued to find means of working together to improve both their individual situations and that of the wider community. Although the project formally came to an end in 1996, some of the hotels continue to organize on their own to this day. Moreover, there are many salutary lessons from this project for professional and voluntary workers alike. As Minkler herself observed:

The message behind this story is a simple one: had students and staff of the Tenderloin Senior Organizing Project failed to pay attention to and support the elders' definition of need – had they not acknowledged, back in the beginning, that crime was indeed a health problem – they might still be running support groups in hotel lobbies one morning a week, if indeed they were still welcome at all. Instead, by trusting the elderly residents to determine and act on their own health agenda, they were able to contribute to something that has had a real and lasting impact on the health of this community.

(Minkler 1996: 476)

Health information and self-care skills: pensioners' health courses (England)

The policy context discussed in Chapter 2, reveals that the 1980s in Britain was a decade littered with various local and national campaigns emphasizing the benefits of sport and exercise, and advocating the adoption of healthy lifestyles for all. However, much of the work during this period was directed at trying to get individuals to change specific aspects of their lifestyles by, for example, dieting or giving up smoking. On the positive side though, these developments did at least draw attention to the fact that older people too were integral to health promotion initiatives.

From among all the activity taking place at that time, this case study has been chosen to detail work carried out by colleagues in the London Borough of Barnet. First, this work clearly illustrates the ways in which it is possible to build on and develop effective activities and support materials from relatively modest beginnings. Second, it highlights the importance of research to our understanding of the roles of professional workers in self health care activities. Finally, the experiences of one of the key workers (Kathy Meade) in these developments was crucial when we later came to work together on the Beth Johnson Foundation's Self Health Care in Old Age Project.

In 1981, the health education unit of the London Borough of Barnet was approached by the local Community Health Council and a voluntary group called Task Force (now Pensioners' Link), to help initiate a health course for older people. As a result, eight older people joined forces with two health and community workers to plan a 12-week course. The course was designed to provide local older people with information about how their bodies work, about their rights and services, and with details of particular medical conditions. The course included sessions on:

- ageing
- bones, backs and joints
- blood pressure and heart conditions
- bowels and waterworks
- diet
- hospital stays
- yoga and relaxation.

All the sessions were designed to challenge the negative expectations surrounding the health of older people. Information sheets were available for course participants to take away with them, and relevant books from the local library were on hand for people to borrow. The success of the courses was due, in large part, to the involvement of older people from the very beginning: to a commitment to working *with* them as opposed to providing a course *for* them. From widely publicized open meetings, pensioner committees were elected which, with the back-up of local workers, oversaw the courses, planned the programme details, and made all the arrangements concerning speakers, venues, publicity, and transport for housebound older people. This not only ensured that the topics covered were relevant to the needs and interests of older people, but also meant that the motivation and interest generated longer-term developments.

As a result of the success of the first course, additional groups of older people across the borough worked together with other professionals to set up their own courses. No two courses were the same, and the range of topics covered was extensive. The courses also triggered a variety of follow-up activities. For example, three thriving social activity clubs developed which incorporated keep-fit and relaxation groups, and regular health issues discussion sessions. Elsewhere, a swimming club and a lip-reading class were established, and other health groups were also begun. Existing groups and organizations were also stimulated to include health education sessions in their regular social activities. It is evident, therefore, that by actively involving older people from the outset in the planning and development of courses, this can have longer term beneficial spin-offs.

In 1985, Barnet Pensioners' Link received funding from the Health Education Council for a two-year project aimed at consolidating this earlier work. Kathy Meade's initial task was to review the work already undertaken and to research the experiences of those who had participated in the health courses. Between May and July 1985, 187 older people, 19 speakers and 14 group coordinators completed questionnaires. The main findings from this research highlight a number of key issues concerning the role of professional workers in the development of courses designed to promote self health care activities among older people (Meade 1986). These include:

- The importance of involving older people in planning the course content, both in general terms and in relation to individual topics.
- The need to challenge the traditional pattern of health education for older people, which mostly consists of one-off talks on broad topics, given in didactic fashion to large groups.
- The importance of properly briefing speakers about the interests, needs and knowledge levels of the particular group.
- The need for adequate time to be built in so that ideas and information can be shared, and so that participants can also have 'private chats' with speakers if they wish.
- The provision of good teaching aids and of leaflets for people to take away and read at their own leisure.

The workers and group coordinators also recognized the importance of their role as enablers, but were aware that the process of actively involving the 'consumers' in decision-making processes is often slower and more complex than at first anticipated. Time then is crucial: time to nurture the development and to respond to any longer term initiatives that emerge.

Finally, it was evident that promoting self health care by such means is often something that is squeezed in around other commitments, and has often not been accepted as a legitimate part of many health professionals' jobs. Clearly then, it is crucially important for preventive work of this nature to become a recognized priority among a range of professionals involved in helping to sustain the health and well-being of older people, an issue to which we shall return in later chapters.

For the older people, participation in the courses proved to have had many beneficial outcomes. About two-thirds of them had come for the prime reason that they had an interest in keeping themselves healthy, although the chance to make new friends and to go to something which offered more than the traditional game of bingo was also a decided attraction. Many of them made use of the information which was provided and had sought practical help from various services as well as taking steps to maintain or improve their own health. Their understanding and self-confidence was also enhanced, as these comments illustrate (HEC/Age Concern England 1985):

> I think these talks help us because doctors have very little time – they prescribe pills. When we come to these meetings, things are explained to us about illnesses. And we know what to do to look after ourselves.

> I've learnt more about my blood pressure. I've had it for seven years. I've found out what the pills are doing for me.

> The health club's lovely. It brings us out, gets us mixing with people socially – we're making lots of friends.

Arising out of all this work, a 'how to' guide was developed to provide guidelines, activities and resources for people interested in developing health courses with older people (Meade 1987). Five principles underlie the approach taken in the guide, and these clearly echo the self-empowered orientation to health outlined at the close of Chapter 3:

- a belief that older people want to learn more about maintaining and improving their health in later life;
- a recognition that older people themselves have considerable knowledge and valuable experience to share with each other and with health professionals;
- an acknowledgement that older people can take positive steps both to improve their own health and to prevent illness;
- a commitment to involve older people at every stage in the planning of self health care activities of whatever kind;
- an appreciation that an individual's health is influenced not only by their own attitudes but also by the political, social and economic worlds in which they live.

The guide is intended for use in a variety of settings, and in the hope and expectation that many more older people will be enabled to gain the information, skills and support which they require in order to promote their own health and well-being to the best of their abilities.

Peer support, research and development: Century House (Canada)

Century House is a seniors' recreation centre located in the city of New Westminster in the Province of British Columbia. Modelled after similar projects in the United States, this first senior centre of its kind in Canada was opened by Princess Margaret in 1959; 40 years later it had over 2100 members. Although it began life as a project designed to serve the leisure needs of older people, Century House has, over the years, broadened its remit to encompass related areas. In particular, in the 1980s Century House developed a senior peer counselling service, a programme that trains older people to assist others in the community to lead more positive lifestyles. Century House has also worked closely with the Gerontology Research Centre at nearby Simon Fraser University in Vancouver, and this collaboration is evidenced in a variety of research and development projects directed towards lifelong learning and education, including the Mental Fitness Programme described below.

I have been fortunate since the mid-1980s to meet and correspond with a number of key personnel associated with these developments, including Beryl Petty, who served as trainer/consultant to the senior peer counselling programme in the 1980s and continues in this capacity to the present day. Beryl, along with Sandra Cusack, currently a research associate at the Gerontology Research Centre, documented the effectiveness of Century House's peer counselling programme (Petty and Cusack 1989). In 1993, Dr Cusack and Wendy Thompson, the Seniors' Wellness Coordinator for the Simon Fraser Health Region, were employed by Century House to train a group of seniors as researchers, and to assist them in conducting an assessment of the lifelong learning needs of the membership. Among the results, it was evident that older people felt that 'mental fitness' was just as important as physical fitness and that the brain needed to continue to be exercised and developed as well as the body.

With further funding, a second research and development study attempted to expand the role of seniors by developing a group of mental fitness advocates, working with them to explore and define the concept more closely, and then producing a mental fitness pilot programme. The goal of this project was, and still is, to establish mental fitness as an essential component of an holistic approach to healthy ageing. The three phases of the initial project – planning and promotion, research and development, and evaluation and strategic planning – spanned a six-month period. Following a series of planning sessions with a steering committee comprising the director and programmer of Century House, the centre's Lifelong Learning Advisory Group and an adult education coordinator, advertisements were placed in the centre's newsletter and in a local newspaper, inviting interested participants to an introductory session.

Thirty-eight people aged between 55 and 84 (average age 73) who attended the first session agreed to become part of a research team which would meet for a series of weekly sessions for one afternoon a week over six weeks. The intention in these weekly focus group sessions was that participants would review readings from the literature on ageing and mental health and contribute their own articles, knowledge and experience to discussion and debate. Through a grounded theory approach, these discussions would then be translated into the components of a mental fitness programme. Participants completed a preliminary questionnaire which yielded basic socio-demographic data, but which also asked about people's mental functioning, how they would define 'mental fitness' and what their concerns and fears were. Using these data, the group began to address the issues through discussions, games, puzzles and other small group tasks. Arising out of this, the group generated a list of issues which they felt needed to be addressed in a mental fitness programme:

- memory
- infirmities and health problems
- a forum for sharing for people who live alone
- inability to continue learning serious topics and technology
- not to be set in my ways, or averse to change
- to be positive and willing to learn
- loss of independence
- loss of mental functioning
- fears that I won't measure up
- meeting new people and doing new things
- attitudes of people
- being deadwood
- being criticized for expressing opinions
- speaking in public.

They also wrestled with defining the concept of mental fitness, and trying to explain its relationship with healthy ageing. Some comments from the summary report (Cusack and Thompson 1995) are illustrative:

> Mental fitness is having the ability to retain an open mind, learning to cope.

> I keep wanting to compare mental fitness to physical fitness. You go to a physical fitness class to get in shape – then you join a tennis club. We need to work on our mind muscles.

> Mental fitness means thinking positively; believing in our own capabilities; setting goals; and being able to change as the situation arises.

> Mental fitness promotes healthy aging by providing the tools and the confidence to take responsibility for physical health.
>
> (Cusack and Thompson 1995: 19–20)

From these deliberations, reflections, small group activities and lively debates, the consultants drafted a programme outline which was then presented to the group for further discussion and adaptation. The agreed pilot programme – a series of eight all-day intensive workshops – was run at

Century House towards the end of 1996. The outline programme was presented as follows:

A MENTAL FITNESS PROGRAM FOR SENIORS

Mental Fitness is vital to healthy aging and it encompasses a number of abilities/skills that can be developed. Like physical fitness, it is a condition of optimal functioning that is achieved through regular exercise and a healthy lifestyle. Mental Fitness includes creative thinking, clear thinking, problem-solving, memory skills, learning new things, and expressing ideas clearly. Seniors tell us that it also includes setting personal goals and developing positive mental attitudes such as:

- optimism (as opposed to fearfulness)
- confidence (as opposed to timidity)
- flexibility (as opposed to rigidity)
- self-esteem (as opposed to low self-worth)
- a willingness to risk (as opposed to playing it safe)

INTRODUCTION TO MENTAL FITNESS

An eight-week course for adults 50+ to exercise your mental muscles presented as a series of workshops.

SESSION 1: Introduction
SESSION 2: Clear thinking
SESSION 3: Problem-solving
SESSION 4: Learning new things
SESSION 5: Creative thinking
SESSION 6: Memory skills
SESSION 7: Expressing ideas clearly
SESSION 8: Goal setting

As we explore these aspects of mental fitness, the focus will be on:

- enlightening and lightening up – i.e. having more fun
- building self-esteem and confidence
- developing open-mindedness and flexibility
- challenging people to take risks
- stimulating the desire to continue to learn and grow

Eighteen people (fifteen women and three men) between the ages of 63 and 83 registered for the first course, and a variety of methods were used to evaluate the extent to which it achieved its objectives. These included pre and post-course questionnaires; a participant observation record of all sessions; take-home questions for participants; and focus group discussions. During the course, participants learnt how attitudes and beliefs about the mental abilities of older people restricted their options for leading a productive and rewarding old age. They learnt how to change and modify their beliefs and behaviours and how to avoid using limiting language. They also listened to each other with respect and consideration, and learnt how to appreciate differing perspectives and diverse views.

The evaluation of the pilot programme (Cusack and Thompson 1996) demonstrated that participants had gained from their involvement in a number of respects. All reported dramatic increases in their level of mental fitness and many improved their memory. Others noted changes in their attitudes and as the course progressed participants appeared visibly more positive, confident and relaxed. Beliefs and behaviours were also affected with every participant achieving a goal they had set for themselves (such as losing weight, quitting smoking or completing a particular project such as a painting). Two comments from participants encapsulate these changes:

> I used to believe that old age meant gradual decline in body and mind, and that I had to learn to accept my limitations in an uncomplaining way and look for the joy in nature and those things that endure. Now I believe that no matter what the future holds, there will be new goals and activities to challenge my mind and abilities.

> I have a newfound energy that is enabling me to think more clearly. I am doing things I never thought I could because of this excitement I have. I am striving for things I never thought I could achieve. Perhaps it was the limiting beliefs that held me back.

This pilot project was completed in 1997 with two follow-up sessions for the inaugural group and a series of half-day workshops designed to introduce new people to mental fitness. With funding from the Seniors' Health Promotion Network, senior leaders from Century House continue to work as mental fitness advocates speaking to groups and individuals around British Columbia. In recognition of this research and development project, Century House received the 1997 Research Award presented annually by the Washington-based National Institute of Seniors Centers (NISC). Because Canada does not have an equivalent national organization, this was a particular honour for Century House and brought both recognition and renewed impetus to the work they had been doing for 40 years.

For the future, it is the desire of the consultants to be able to replicate this development in other contexts and with other groups in different countries. They believe that this approach, which they have dubbed 'research as emancipatory education' (Cusack 1998), offers a way of empowering older people not solely through self-help or mutual aid, but also by drawing on and utilizing the skills of adult educators and educational gerontologists in a constructive and mutually beneficial enterprise.

Reaching out: the CHAYIL 'Add Life to Years' Project (Israel)

For many decades now, the World Health Organization has been active in promoting the health of older people. The Health for All policy incorporates healthy ageing as one of its key targets, and much work is being undertaken through the auspices of what are known as WHO Collaborating Centres. One such centre is the JDC Brookdale Institute of Gerontology and Human Development in Jerusalem which is evaluating a new health promotion programme aimed at meeting the diverse needs of elderly people in Israel.

Begun in 1992, the CHAYIL project is based on North American self health care models. Adapted from the City of New York's Stay Well health promotion programme, it focuses on training 'young' elderly people to promote health among their peers. CHAYIL – the Hebrew acronym for 'Add Life to Years' – is run and funded at a national level by Eshel, the Association for the Planning and Development of Services for the Elderly in Israel. Its activities are overseen by a director of health promotion, while local coordinators are employed in each location served by the programme.

CHAYIL began in the towns of Kfar Saba, Rehovot and Ramat Gan, and has been extended to Karmiel, a town with a high proportion of recent immigrants, many of them from the former Soviet Union; to the large metropolitan area of Tel Aviv; and to the rural area of Shaar Hanegev, which includes a total of thirteen scattered kibbutzim (communal villages). The variation in locations means that although CHAYIL is organized around a common core training programme, the activities engaged in by volunteers must respond very much to the local situation. Volunteer recruitment is the responsibility of the local coordinators. They target 'new pensioners', often by obtaining lists of retirees from workplaces, by word of mouth and through local publicity. Volunteers are screened and they are expected to have positive attitudes towards health and to be actively involved in community life. They then undergo formal training in their own locality. This training consists of a thirteen-session course, undertaken over three months and led by professionals. The course covers:

- memory
- hearing problems and their treatment
- vision problems and their treatment
- communication with medical staff
- proper use of medication
- sleeping problems and solutions
- prevention of falls and accidents in the home
- road safety
- care of the feet
- correct body posture and movement
- sensible nutrition
- oral and dental hygiene
- physical activity.

On completion of the course, volunteers assist local coordinators to run a range of health promotion activities for other older people. By 1995, 180 people between the ages of 53 and 75 had participated in the six training courses run in each locality. The evaluation shows that volunteers are predominantly middle-class 'young elderly' women (83 per cent), with an average age of 68.5 years. Half were European-American born, one-third were Israeli born, a minority (14 per cent) were Asian-African born, and 2 per cent were from the former Soviet Union. Most had migrated to Israel prior to the establishment of the state in 1948. The majority (85 per cent) had retired from work and volunteered in other spheres as well (71 per cent); 86 per cent of them were physically active themselves, maintaining a healthy lifestyle through activities such as swimming, walking and exercising. Only 4 per cent of the volunteers smoked.

The roles of volunteers develop and expand in response to both the desires and capabilities of the individual volunteer, as well as the differing needs and challenges posed by each locality. The main kinds of activities in which volunteers have been involved include

- running health promotion discussion groups in homes for elderly people, in day care centres and in senior clubs (in 1996, for example, 35 such groups were held involving 1156 participants);
- organizing and leading activity groups such as walking clubs (these usually take place once or twice a week);
- assisting professionals in screening for hearing and visual problems in community clinics and senior clubs, and conducting follow-up visits and treatments (in 1996, 1063 people had hearing tests and 754 vision tests);
- holding discussion groups on safety and hazards in the home, and engaging in screening for environmental risk factors in people's own homes;
- setting up and maintaining 'Chayil Corners' in local public libraries;
- organizing, with the coordinator, health fairs.

Eshel provides ongoing training on specific subjects, and there are also additional day seminars, together with the provision of written and audiovisual materials to assist volunteers in their counselling and group leadership roles. CHAYIL attempts to develop a corporate and ideological identity among its volunteers and participants, by enrolling them all as members and having identity cards, a logo, tee shirts and hats. In addition to the trained volunteers, who currently number about 350, it is estimated that about 3000 older people have been involved in CHAYIL activities.

An indication of the need to reach out in a flexible manner to other older people comes from examining the development of groups in differing locations. In the town of Ramat Gan, for example, the walking groups proved to be extremely popular while in Rehovot, volunteers discovered that older people really preferred to walk alone. Similarly, the health concerns and needs of urban and rural elderly people were found to differ markedly. The kibbutzim of the Shaar Hanegev area are, like many kibbutzim in Israel, coming to terms with the move away from a totally collective lifestyle to a more individualized lifestyle. The elderly kibbutz member who had been used to eating in the communal dining room for the past fifty years is now faced with learning anew how to manage an individual budget, buying and preparing food. Nutrition programmes here are, consequently, faced with different issues from nutritional programmes for elderly people in the urban areas.

Eshel monitors, supports and funds the CHAYIL programme. It provides guidance to a steering group of local coordinators, fully funds the programmes in each area for the first year of operation, pays for 75 per cent in the second year, and then only for volunteer training in the third year. From the third year, programmes are funded from local budgets. In other words, the longer term aim is that programmes at the local level are essentially self-funding after the initial two-year start-up period. This means that local coordinators have a major networking task to perform with possible funding agencies in their areas, in order to establish and maintain an independent infrastructure after Eshel withdraws its financial support.

Aside from Eshel's monitoring function, an external monitoring and evaluation of the project is being carried out by the Brookdale Institute in Jerusalem. This evaluation is formative in nature and is being used to feed back and modify elements of the programme as it progresses. For example, evaluation of the first training course led to modifications to the second, and so on. Evaluation also highlighted the need for some practical training to complement the theoretical orientation of the course. As a result, previously trained volunteer group leaders now meet up with new recruits, and practical sessions on group leadership and group dynamics have been introduced in order to boost the volunteers' self-confidence in what they are doing. Subjective self-reports from volunteers suggest that participation in the training programmes has been beneficial to them in a number of ways. Knowledge levels have increased, attitudes towards the value of health promotion have become more positive, and volunteers report improvements in their physical and mental health status, and in their social situations. The evaluation is also looking at the organizational infrastructure, and at the degree of cooperation among the various agencies involved in the project. This is particularly important because CHAYIL aims to complement, not supplant, existing services.

As with many projects of this nature, monitoring and evaluation is extremely complex. The variability and dynamism of the project means that it does not lend itself to highly structured or rigid kinds of evaluation. It is also very reliant on the cooperation of the elderly volunteers in terms of data collection. While many are seemingly happy to fill in monitoring sheets such as attendance forms for particular activities, getting them to evaluate what has occurred appears to be more difficult. The researchers are therefore having to experiment with other less intrusive or potentially threatening ways of evaluating activities, including observation of activities and questionnaires administered to participants. These difficulties are not unique, as we shall see in Chapter 5. Rather, they illustrate just how reflexive and sensitive research needs to be when it is trying to capture such important changes to the health and well-being of older individuals and the communities in which they live.

Conclusion

From these brief case studies, we can see that they share a number of features which are common to the development of projects and programmes aimed at enhancing the health and well-being of older people. They also illustrate the scope of activity and research which self health care now encompasses. However, rather than delineating these attributes here we shall turn first to the details of the Beth Johnson Foundation's Self Health Care in Old

Age Project. Then, in the light of all these discussions, we shall return, in the final chapter, to the range of lessons we can usefully learn from these action research projects in order to articulate the role which self health care might fulfil in future policy and practice affecting older people.

5

Self health care in practice:
the Self Health Care in
Old Age Project

Introduction

The first half of this book has been devoted to a broad overview of the place of self health care in the overall context of health policy and health promotion. With this as a background, we turn now to a detailed consideration of one particular programme first developed in Britain during the latter half of the 1980s: the Beth Johnson Foundation's Self Health Care in Old Age Project. This chapter presents a brief historical résumé of the local, national and international contexts in which the project was developed, and details its four main elements: peer health counselling, CareLine (a telephone link service), health-related courses and activities, and the Senior Health Shop. The chapter concludes with a consideration of the funding, staffing and managerial aspects of the project.

The local context

Before discussing the elements of the project in detail, it is important to sketch in a little about the sponsoring organization, the Beth Johnson Foundation. The project did not emerge out of the blue; on the contrary, it evolved from many years' work and involvement with older people, and was established in response to the needs and wishes which they themselves were expressing. In this sense, the Self Health Care in Old Age Project was very much a community development/action research project in its fullest sense.

Located in Stoke-on-Trent in North Staffordshire, the Beth Johnson Foundation is a charitable trust set up in 1972 following the death of Mrs Beth Johnson. Her will provided for the whole of her estate to be used for charitable purposes, and the Foundation was established as a memorial to her. Unusually for a charitable organization, it was decided very early on that instead of adopting a conventional welfarism approach, perhaps through the disbursement of sums of money to help 'poor and needy' older people, the Foundation would aim to sponsor and encourage a variety of innovative work. Its main aim has been to improve the quality of life of older people through practical initiatives, research and evaluation (both in-house and for outside organizations) and educational activities. It has always operated with a very small core staff. In 1982, when I was appointed on a temporary one-year contract as research officer, I joined a full-time director and a development officer, plus two administrative staff. Thus, from its earliest days, the Foundation's activities have always been reliant on sources of external funding as a complement to its own financial resources. The projects that it establishes have had to work towards becoming self-supporting within a comparatively short time span (usually two to three years), in order that the core staff can move on and develop new activities.

Early developments

During the 1970s, the Foundation sponsored the development of various projects for older people. Some of these might now be considered as fairly conventional – an over-60s day centre in the middle of the largest council housing estate in the city (Johnson 1979a); a mobile day centre serving the needs of elderly people living in rural areas of Staffordshire (Johnson 1979b); and neighbourhood support schemes for mentally infirm older people and their carers (Bernard 1983, 1984a; Bernard *et al.* 1983). Set in its historical context, some of these developments were early examples of pioneering work with older people.

The Foundation was responsible, in 1976, for establishing one of the first housing associations aimed at meeting the needs of this sector of the population. The Beth Johnson Housing Association (as it was then called) was responsible for building and managing a variety of sheltered housing schemes. Although constitutionally, physically and financially separate, the Beth Johnson Housing Group (as it is now) retains strong links with the Foundation, but has developed a wider remit for social housing aimed at meeting the needs of other client groups.

During the 1980s, there was a discernible shift of emphasis in the Foundation's work, as the early developments gathered momentum and the staff were able to encourage and support new projects based increasingly on peer and self-help. In 1982, for example, the Beth Johnson Leisure Association came into being. This still-flourishing organization, with some 800 members currently, was concerned with opening up local opportunities for older people to engage in sporting and other recreational activities, and now provides a regular programme of sports and social activities across North Staffordshire (Bernard 1984b). Now independent of the Foundation, it is managed by the members and the range of activities on offer are led, for the most part, by older people themselves.

Hot on the heels of the Leisure Association came the Beth Johnson Senior

Centre. Opened in 1983 and originally located in a converted city centre church, it is now accommodated in club premises belonging to a different church, and offers a wide range of both sedentary and energetic activities, as well as refreshments and meals. It also provides older people with the opportunity to make new social contacts, to learn new skills and to seek advice which they might need. Again, older people run most of the activities themselves and serve in a voluntary capacity in the preparation of food.

Health and well-being in old age

One of the most striking features arising out of these early developments was the keen interest exhibited by many older people in maintaining their own health. A course on first aid in the home, held at the Senior Centre in early 1984, proved to be particularly popular. Around this time too, the Foundation began to work with the Centre for Health and Retirement Education (CHRE) based in London. Three health issues discussion groups were established, exploring a range of concerns related to health in retirement, and trying out materials being developed for use on pre-retirement courses.

The first group was drawn from participants in the first aid course. In common with many older people, their worst fears centred around being unable to look after themselves, and becoming increasingly dependent on others. This was countered, however, by an equally strong desire and resolve to stay as fit and active as possible, and to learn as much as they could about remaining healthy. Many of this group went on to take part later that year in a Staying Healthy in Retirement course, led jointly by the Foundation's development officer and by a health education officer from the health authority. Twenty one people joined the course. At the first session, participants identified areas of particular interest and these were then followed up with the help of professional workers during subsequent weeks. The original ten-session course thus expanded into a five-month programme.

During this time, participants covered topics as diverse as first aid; diet and nutrition; movement and mobility; stress management; care of the feet; chronic illness; alternative medicine; emotional adjustments and confidence building; bereavement, loss and other later life crises. Women participants dominated and although one or two men attended some of the sessions, they were very reluctant to participate, particularly when discussions were concerned with feelings and emotions. At one session, the women graphically described how chatting and gossiping was, for them, a useful way of alleviating worry, anxiety and depression. They felt that retirement, with its loss of workmates, was particularly difficult because it often deprived them of this means of communication. In stark contrast, the three men present felt that this strategy was never really available to them. As a consequence, they would carry their worries and anxieties with them, with adverse effects on their well-being (Ivers 1985).

The second health issues discussion group comprised a number of the active swimmers and ramblers from the Leisure Association. Not surprisingly, they were very health conscious and of the strong opinion that people should be encouraged to be active much earlier in life. They were unequivocal about the need for professionals to stop labelling them as 'old', for GPs to stop talking down to them, and for teachers and providers to break away from the view that education is just for the young. They wanted to be recognized and appreciated for what they too had to offer, but were also aware of the need for, and value of, mutual aid and support.

The third discussion group consisted of older unemployed people. As a group, they were the most acutely aware of the close link between their feelings and emotions, and their sense of health and well-being. Their particular concerns centred around personal status, relationships and mental health, and they strongly demonstrated the immense value and importance of being able to talk such issues through in the supportive company of their peers. Participants in these three discussion groups also made a number of very pertinent comments about the ways in which health and well-being might be promoted among older people. For example, they observed that: 'What we need is somewhere to go when we're well; somewhere to ask about anything that is worrying you, where you can chat over the little things'. They were also of the opinion that: 'We ourselves have to encourage other people to come and join us'.

The seeds of the Self Health Care in Old Age Project

By listening carefully to these people, and to the wider constituencies represented through the Leisure Association and the Senior Centre, it became increasingly evident to Foundation staff that conventional health education, while addressing certain needs, was clearly missing others. It was apparent that there was considerable scope for extending the skills and abilities of the many 'natural helpers' with whom we had contact – the older people who were already working with us as volunteers in various capacities. Specifically, we became increasingly concerned with how we might enable and support older people to be a positive resource for their peers.

In 1985, and again in partnership with the Centre for Health and Retirement Education, we instigated the first British-based pilot peer counselling course. On a study visit to the United States, the Foundation's development officer had visited a project in Santa Monica, California, where trained older volunteers provided community support to other older people by promoting healthy lifestyles, encouraging people to take up exercise and modify their diet, detecting any changes in health status, and by generally improving morale. On her return, she felt that such a project would fit very well with the directions in which the Foundation's developments were moving. Consequently, it was decided to offer older people the opportunity to participate in a training programme to equip them with some basic skills, provide them with more information about local services and facilities, and to begin to develop a counselling approach to health-related work with their peers.

The ten-session training course, held between January and June 1985, comprised two introductory sessions (in January and February), a six-session residential weekend (in March) and two follow-up sessions (in May and June). Led jointly by the Foundation's development officer and a member of the CHRE, and monitored by the Foundation's research officer, the course was designed to enable older volunteers to lead groups of other older people in health-related discussions and activities, or to engage in individual coun-selling and support work with their peers (Bernard and Ivers 1986; Ivers and Meade 1991). This pilot Peer Health Counselling course and the work which followed from it, proved to be the immediate forerunner of the much larger Self Health Care in Old Age Project.

The national context

As we saw in Chapter 2, the first half of the 1980s was also a time when the then Health Education Council was developing its Health in Old Age Pro-gramme. Launched in the spring of 1985, it was the first national British pro-gramme of its kind. Ambitious though the plan was, the scale of it was fairly modest, especially when set alongside the kinds of activities and expenditure devoted to curative, hospital-based services. However, it did contribute to an emerging consciousness among many organizations of the tremendous need and potential to enhance the health and well-being of older adults. For the Beth Johnson Foundation (hereafter referred to as 'the Foundation'), the pro-gramme was another piece in the developmental jigsaw which we had been carefully constructing since the early 1980s. It also seemed, at the time, that the programme might provide us with a means of possible co-funding for the further development of our activities.

In anticipation of the Health in Old Age Programme and the Age Well cam-paign, the Foundation put together a bid for a demonstration project entitled Self Health Care in Old Age (Creber *et al.* 1985). The focus of the bid was on health promotion and education, and it detailed various sets of developmental activities:

• an 'Age Well' Health Counselling Centre
• an outreach counselling scheme
• a telephone link scheme
• the production of information and training packs
• a training programme for professionals and volunteers
• comprehensive research and evaluation.

Unfortunately, our attempts to secure co-funding through the national pro-gramme were unsuccessful. Despite the overall aim of the programme noted above, it had become increasingly evident in our discussions with the HEC that certain officers in the funding body (the DHSS) were still sceptical about the particular value of developing self health care activities with older people. It was also proving difficult within the HEC itself to link this aspect of health education to an overall national strategy. For the Foundation, the timing of the HEC programme eventually proved to be inappropriate: we were keen to press on with our developments at precisely the time when the HEC decided to devote its first two-year phase to the collation and dissemination of good practice. Direct financial support for projects was a future possibility but not a present reality. Clearly then, even in the mid-1980s, there was a seeming reluctance on the part of 'government' to support such peer and self-help activities generated by a charitable trust, as opposed to enhancing profes-sionally led health education.

The European context

Quite fortuitously, however, the Foundation was advised by Age Concern England of wider European developments. In December 1984, the European Economic Community's Council of Ministers formally agreed to make financial provision for a Second Programme to Combat Poverty in member states. It was expected that resources of about £12 million would be made available, and that the UK might attract about one-fifth of this amount.

The second programme was partly based on recommendations arising from its predecessor, which ran from 1975 to 1980. By the mid-1980s, the European Community was confronted with approximately 30 million of its citizens living in poverty. In response, 25 million ECU (1 European Currency Unit = £0.60 approx at 1984 levels) were allocated to finance a four-year programme aimed at combining research with innovatory projects, addressing issues of common application to the then ten member states. The programme was to be focused on eight different target groups:

* long-term unemployed people
* young unemployed people
* elderly people
* single parent families
* migrants
* marginal groups
* underprivileged people in urban areas
* underprivileged people in rural areas.

To be eligible for funding, certain other ground rules had also to be satisfied. These included:

* *Action research* – proposals had to show that they had monitoring and evaluation built into them, whether internally or externally.
* *Location* – projects had to be sited in 'deprived urban' or 'impoverished rural' areas.
* *Special features* – among other things, the European Commission was interested in projects that could clearly demonstrate how they would alleviate poverty; how people would effectively participate in activities; how it would fit with local, regional and national developments; and how evaluation and dissemination would be carried out.

Furthermore, with respect to the target group of elderly people, the Commission recognized that 'the poverty that impoverishes the lives of elderly people (who constitute over 40 million people in the EEC), is often not a direct cause of economic factors, such as inadequate income, but due to a poverty of access to health care, or companionship, for example' (Animation and Dissemination Service 1985: 2).

With this in mind, five areas of action were identified, where it was hoped that projects might contribute to the alleviation of poverty among older people:

* *Education and recreation* – whereby elderly people would be introduced to new opportunities, and encouraged to teach and pass on their skills in particular activities.

- *Health and community care* – to promote the philosophy of community care, to support elderly people to stay in their own homes for as long as possible, and to encourage links between forms of 'institutional' care and the wider community.
- *Housing* – to maintain, upgrade and adapt existing dwellings and to promote experimental group living projects.
- *Benefits* – to encourage and facilitate the take-up of benefits to which elderly people are entitled.
- *Elderly minorities* – in recognition of the diverse make-up of the group labelled 'elderly people'.

In the UK, the DHSS was to be responsible for the programme and, in the spring of 1985, proposals for funding were invited from both statutory and voluntary agencies. The European Commission would meet 50 per cent of the total for projects costing in the region of £50,000 to £100,000 each.

Evidently, the Foundation's existing and proposed developments appeared to dovetail quite readily with some of the major thrusts of the poverty programme: elderly people were a key target group; there was an emphasis on health, education and recreational activities, and on the development of peer help and support; our 'locality' was impoverished and in receipt at that time of other kinds of urban aid; and the programme was oriented around an action research model. Consequently, Foundation staff moved quickly to put together a modified bid. This bid proved successful and, in December 1985, the Foundation and the European Commission agreed a contract for the work.

Thus, with funding secured, and against a background of both national and European developments around these issues, we turn now to consider the elements of the Self Health Care in Old Age Project in greater detail.

The Self Health Care in Old Age Project: its philosophical and conceptual basis

The historical development of the Foundation's activities reveals that, certainly by the 1980s, notions of empowerment, peer and self-help were key organizing principles of the work. These features were explicitly brought together under the umbrella of the Self Health Care in Old Age Project. While the project has obviously evolved and changed since its inception in 1986, its overall aims and objectives still remain firmly rooted in the idea of self-empowered health behaviour, as outlined at the end of Chapter 3.

A focus on 'empowerment' suggests that people are, by definition, in situations where they feel 'powerless'. Indeed, in the context of the European Poverty Programme, it was incumbent upon the Foundation to demonstrate the ways in which our project would address the needs of 'poor' elderly people. Objectively speaking, this project, like many of the Foundation's earlier activities, was directed at older people from lower socio-economic groups. Its proposed location, in the commercial and business centre of Stoke-on-Trent (in Hanley), also meant that it would draw heavily on the population in the immediate vicinity. Data about this population revealed that there was a higher than average proportion of elderly people in the locality, living mainly in the small streets of terraced housing which still border the city centre. Traditionally too, women have formed a substantial part of the workforce in North Staffordshire, working predominantly in the pottery industry. The largest employer of men was, until relatively recently, the National Coal Board, together with one or two other large factories, including tyre manufacture. Additionally, ownership and access to a car, especially among older people, tended to be lower than average, though the city centre itself was fairly well served by public transport.

In addition to these 'objective' measures of poverty, it was important to the project to adopt a broader definition than one based solely on indicators of income or wealth (Piachaud 1987). Following Townsend (1987), we felt that it was more helpful to conceptualize poverty in much wider terms, to include social, cultural and political dimensions, as well as financial aspects. This is encapsulated in the notion of 'deprivation', defined by Townsend (1987: 125) as 'a state of observable and demonstrable disadvantage relative to the local community or the wider society or nation'. This notion of deprivation was further subdivided into two categories: material deprivation and social deprivation.

We further argued that older adults, like all people, can be said to be deprived if they lack the means to live, for example, in acceptable housing or to eat an adequate diet. They can also be said to be deprived if they do not have access to, or are unable to participate in, forms of recreation, education, occupation, social and health care opportunities commonly available in our society. If people are denied the resources they need to attain these material and social conditions, they can be said to be 'in poverty'. Such poverty tends to exclude and marginalize people, and involves loss of power, choice and control over one's life. It also leads to a sense of isolation and segregation arising in part from not having the material means to participate in community life, but also from being conscious of being excluded from, but not immune to, the pressures of a consumer society (Robbins 1987b). Exclusion of older people in these ways is also about our attitudes towards them, and about the self-concepts that older people hold about themselves. Alongside their exclusion and segregation often go feelings of a lack of confidence, of self-esteem or self-worth – all issues which it was hoped our project would begin to address.

Thus, in the context of our work with older people in the project, we defined poverty as 'a function of social exclusion from, or denial of access to, the kinds of information, knowledge, social contact, recreational, educational and health care opportunities which might enhance well-being in later years' (Bernard 1988: 87). Furthermore, by orienting the project around a model of self-empowered health behaviour, it was hoped that we would be able to assist individuals to increasingly take charge of themselves and their lives and, by so doing, to become a positive resource for their peers. With this as the conceptual and philosophical context, what did the project look like in practice?

The project in action

The project officially commenced at the beginning of 1986. Its main aim was 'to provide an accessible, attractive and popular means of furthering health education and promotion among older people'. Underlying this aim were three main principles which between them echoed the self-empowerment factors discussed in Chapter 3:

- to raise older people's awareness of the need for health care and maintenance;
- to encourage the involvement of more older people in health care programmes;
- to assist older people to identify their health needs, and to develop the skills and strategies they require to obtain the resources to meet their needs.

In order to achieve these aims and objectives, four main interrelated areas of activity have been developed:

- a Peer Health Counselling scheme
- CareLine – a telephone link service
- health-related courses and activities
- the Senior Health Shop.

Each of these is now briefly discussed in turn, before considering how the project as a whole has been funded, staffed and managed.

Peer Health Counselling

Having secured funding, the pilot Peer Health Counselling scheme was integrated into the wider project and subsequently expanded and developed. Following the success of the initial training course, an annual recruitment drive has ensured that new cohorts of volunteers have come into the scheme each year. The 1985 group of eleven counsellors have been joined by similar-sized groups in subsequent years, though the basic structure of the training has remained fairly constant. It consists of two main elements:

- a three-day induction/initial training course (originally residential but not always so);
- a regular programme of counsellor support and training.

Specific details of the training can be found in Ivers and Meade (1991), while results from the monitoring and evaluation will be discussed in succeeding chapters. In outline, recruitment and training are considered to be especially important for the Foundation's volunteers. People who respond to the recruitment drive are all contacted and given details about the scheme, the training and the commitment expected of them. It is vital that potential volunteers are enabled to make real choices about whether or not this kind of activity will really suit them. If they decide to proceed, each person is interviewed – either in their own home or at the Foundation, as they choose. A detailed form is completed and references taken up.

Following this selection process, two meetings are held prior to the induction course. The main purpose of these meetings is to begin the process of team building and to get to know one another. Volunteers, many of whom are understandably nervous about undertaking 'educational activity', are familiarized with the course content, and practical details are discussed. An

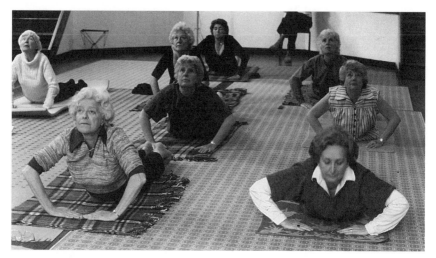

Yoga at the Senior Centre

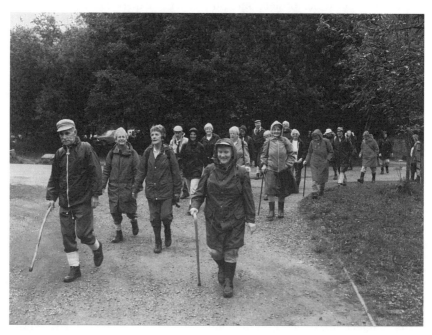

One of the regular rambling groups
© The Beth Johnson Foundation

indication is also given of what might reasonably be expected of participants after the initial training.

The induction course itself comprises a mixture of information-giving sessions together with opportunities for discussion, and the sharing of experiences and skills. The topics cover three main themes: ageing and ageism, positive health in old age, and helping relationships. The aim of these themes is to encourage participants to think critically about their attitudes towards ageing and old age; to explore their beliefs about ageing and health, and to understand the potential for promoting health in later life; and to enhance their listening and responding skills. The course does not train them to become fully fledged counsellors. Rather, it is oriented around a counselling approach, the sharing of information, and the building of self-confidence. In the last session of the course, time is given over to evaluation, to arranging follow-up sessions and to exploring the possible avenues for present and future work.

In addition to the Foundation's development officer, a volunteer support and training officer offers peer health counsellors further training and support at monthly meetings. These sessions build on the residential programme and are tailored to the activities which each counsellor has decided to take on. Old and new counsellors have the opportunity to update each other about what they are doing, and specialist topics, often with a guest speaker, also form part of the sessions. In addition, new counsellors are encouraged to make observation visits – perhaps of half a day each – to a variety of establishments such as homes for elderly people, health clinics, schools, day centres or clubs for older people. They are briefed beforehand, and report back and discuss their impressions at the monthly meetings. They also carry out work on case studies dealing with possible projects which might involve peer health counsellors. These include the giving of information, support and advice to older patients in a health centre; becoming an advocate for a frail elderly person; stimulating activity in a residential home; and engaging older people in reminiscence activities in homes and hospitals.

Peer health counsellors have, and continue to be, involved in a variety of activities including:

- *individual counselling* and support to help people (re)establish their confidence and to (re)introduce them to healthy lifestyle practices such as diet, exercise and stress management strategies;
- *group work* in institutional settings (homes, sheltered housing complexes, day centres) leading gentle exercise, relaxation and health discussion groups;
- *information giving* at health fairs, exhibitions and conferences;
- *advocacy work* with frail older people in hospital settings and in residential and nursing homes;
- *reminiscence therapy*, in partnership with the local museum and library services, in a variety of different settings.

Peer health counsellors are also involved in helping to run the second element of the Self Health Care in Old Age Project, the telephone link scheme.

CareLine – a telephone link service

CareLine, or the Counselling At Risk Elderly telephone service, is aimed at frail, housebound older people. It is a service in which volunteer counsellors maintain regular telephone contact with people deemed to be 'at risk'. Counsellors receive training in telephone counselling techniques, and offer a telephone-out service from Monday to Friday. The service aims to check on the health and well-being of clients, to monitor whether or not they have eaten, slept or taken their prescribed drugs, and to give them some contact with the outside world.

Initially, the service was staffed every afternoon by a counsellor, who phoned up to 25 clients referred to the project by social workers, nurses, health visitors, doctors, carers or relatives. When referrals are made, a member of staff and/or a trained volunteer will visit the potential client to assess whether such a service is truly needed. It is not meant primarily to be a service for those who are lonely, but for people who may, for example, have recently been discharged from hospital or who are in some way vulnerable. The visitor also checks on practical details such as how accessible the telephone is, and in some instances it has been necessary to arrange for the telephone to be moved. Once accepted onto CareLine, calls are made only on those days when no one else will be contacting the older person. Consequently, some people may receive a call each day, while others may be contacted only once or twice a week.

Each CareLine client has a named key person such as a relative or social worker, who can be contacted in the event that volunteers get no reply from the elderly person. After ringing at half-hourly intervals, the volunteer will call the key person towards the end of the afternoon to ask them to check on the client. If that person cannot be contacted either, community police will, as a final safety net, go and investigate. This option has rarely been used, although it is an important part of the available back-up to the service.

Further crucial back-up comes from project staff. The original CareLine was, and is still, located in a small office at the rear of the Senior Health Shop. This means that the volunteers always have someone available should they require additional help or assistance. A second CareLine has been in operation since the summer of 1989, serving the rural area of Staffordshire Moorlands. Originally set up with the aid of a small grant from the Telethon Trust, this line is run in conjunction with Staffordshire Social Services Department, first from an office located in a residential home for older people, and subsequently from the department's offices in the town of Leek. In this way, staff in the home, and then in the department itself, were able to provide professional back-up for the volunteers.

From the one line/one volunteer per day, the service has thus expanded. The two shop-based lines can monitor up to 40 clients, while the Moorlands service now takes between 20 and 30 clients a day. Volunteers have also been able to meet face-to-face with some of the clients who are well enough to travel. Each Christmas, clients were invited to a Christmas party, with transport, lunch and entertainment provided by staff and volunteers. Occasional summer outings also proved popular and the opportunity to put faces to disembodied voices was welcomed by everyone involved.

Although CareLine could be considered as the hidden face of the project, the regular and friendly contact stimulates an interest in self health care for both the caller and the client. The regularity of conversation serves to over-come the anonymity of the telephone and the detailed records which are kept mean that it is possible to monitor the client's health status quite closely. Other services can then be alerted as necessary. In this way, CareLine is used as a preventive, health promoting service for those for whom self health care in the accepted sense is very difficult to achieve. It is also now being recog-nized by the statutory services and is included as part of community care packages (Granville 1998). However, for more active older people, the project also offers the range of health-related courses and activities detailed below.

Health-related courses and activities

There is little point in encouraging people to adopt healthy lifestyles and to look after their health if there are no facilities available through which to achieve this. Many of the activities on offer through the Self Health Care in Old Age Project are run predominantly via the auspices of the Leisure Association and Senior Centre. A non-membership facility, the Senior Centre is open for four days a week (for many years it operated on only three days) to all people over the age of 50 who can get themselves to the centre. Meals and snacks are prepared on the premises by the centre organizer and a band of older volunteers. The centre organizer is a Foundation employee funded, for the main period of the Self Health Care in Old Age Project, from sources other than the European Commission money (this included three years of funding through the national Opportunities for Volunteering Programme).

All the activities on offer are designed with a health-giving or interest-main-taining element. People come together to enhance their social contact, to keep themselves fit and active, and perhaps to take up new activities on retirement. Physical activities include yoga, dancing classes and tea dances, 'popagility' (keep fit to music) and bowls. These are complemented by art, patchwork, needlework and other craft activities, and by musical and educational activi-ties. Seasonal events, outings to places of interest, trips to the theatre, and the occasional organized holiday also form part of the social programme directed at enhancing the social, physical and mental aspects of health in later life. All of these activities are organized, led and tutored by older people themselves.

In addition to these opportunities, we were able to initiate three specific courses under the project, as a direct result of enquiries and problems pre-sented to peer health counsellors and staff in the Senior Health Shop. The first of these was a Look After Yourself (LAY) course tailored to meet the needs of older people, and tutored initially by a lecturer seconded to the Foundation from a local college of further education. The LAY programme combines a period of physical exercise, with a relaxation session and a discussion group around health issues. The exercise element is tailored to individual needs; par-ticipants are taught to monitor their own condition, and to exercise safely and within their personal capabilities. Such was the success of the initial ten-week course that it has become a regular feature of the Senior Centre programme. Subsequently too, an additional course, requested by 'graduates' of the basic course, was fitted in before the yoga class on a Friday morning. The LAY tutor was able to run two further courses: one on stress management and one on nutrition, although these have been offered only occasionally.

Older people in the locality are able to join in the activities which run under the umbrella of the Leisure Association (a financially and constitutionally independent voluntary organization, but which still receives administrative and professional support and guidance from the Foundation's staff). The two main activities which it offers are graded rambles and swimming – both recreational swimming and swimming lessons. There are usually three rambles for most weeks in the year, of varying degrees of difficulty, involving considerable numbers of older people and organized by volunteer leaders. It is possible to swim at six different venues throughout the week, and to be taught to swim by retired instructors. Badminton, table tennis and bowling are available at certain of the leisure centres used by the association. An energetic social committee organizes a whole range of other social events which, over the years, has included adventure holidays and trips abroad. Most recently, the association developed an additional rambling section entitled KITs (Keep In Touch) for those members who have now become less active but who still like to visit the places where they used to walk, and to be with like-minded and enthusiastic people (Granville 1998).

Aside from this range of 'Foundation' or project activities, peer health counsellors and staff make available material and information on other courses, classes and activities in and around the city. Much of this is housed in the Senior Health Shop, to which we now turn our attention.

The Senior Health Shop

Opened on 1 August 1986, the Senior Health Shop has been the focus for much of the project's activities. It is literally the shop window on the project, and on the other activities linked with it. Sited in Hanley – the main commercial centre for the conurbation of Stoke-on-Trent – it is close to the major shopping precincts, opposite the premises of Radio Stoke, and a five-minute walk away from the central bus station serving the whole of North Staffordshire. This means that it is easily accessible to the many people who call in on their way to or from a shopping trip. It is, however, a ten-minute walk away from the Senior Centre.

Open five days a week (as well as on Saturday mornings for an experimental period during its first year of operation), the shop is easily identified by its red and green striped window with its distinctive apple logo. Though very small, it has a light and attractive interior. In order to encourage older people through the door, the front of the shop is set out as a cafeteria with brightly covered round tables and comfortable chairs. Here, customers can purchase drinks and snacks prepared and served by older volunteers, according to recipes approved by the district health authority's dietician. Recipe leaflets giving details of the most popular dishes are available to take away. Once settled with their refreshments, customers become relaxed enough to take an interest in the comprehensive collection of health literature displayed in racks around the walls. This means that they can browse at their leisure, and take whatever catches their interest or particular need at the time.

In addition, shop staff and peer health counsellors, as well as the volunteers, are on hand to discuss health issues with visitors and to advise on suitable activities, diet and exercise programmes for older people. The intention behind the shop concept was that it would provide a relaxed and informal atmosphere, as far removed as possible from the 'clinical' feel of many health care facilities, in which customers would be sufficiently at ease to be able to enquire about any health concerns they had, or to seek advice. While this has been the case, it is evident too that volunteers and staff have become increasingly skilled at identifying when a customer wants to talk about a problem but is finding it difficult to pluck up the courage to make the first approach.

As a health resource, the shop also offers a variety of other services. For the first two years of its operation, the health authority loaned the shop a computer containing half a dozen health and lifestyle quizzes and programmes which customers could use themselves. This proved a novel means of encouraging people to discuss health issues. Blood pressure checking and weight monitoring services are also available and, over the years of European funding, a variety of professional health workers held 'surgeries' at the shop for a morning or an afternoon, talking with, and answering questions from customers. Diet, dental health, housing, exercise and fitness, chiropody, eye care and hearing have been among the topics considered.

Accessibility, appropriate support and extensive information are the key factors in the shop's continuing operation, and has meant that it has remained the most visible part of the project for many years. During the first nine months, we were able to accommodate individuals or groups wanting to visit the project on an ad hoc basis. However, by March 1987 it was evident that this was proving to be increasingly disruptive to the day-to-day running. We therefore instituted monthly Visit Days for which people were asked to book in advance. These continued for the remainder of the initial funding period.

Further issues

Detailing what the project actually consists of provides only certain information to others who might be interested in learning about its operation. Alongside this, there are also recurrent questions concerning how much it costs; who the people are who actually undertake the day-to-day work; and how the project is organized and managed. The rest of this chapter will look at each of these issues in turn.

Funding the project

The remit of the Poverty Programme allowed for the European Commission to fund only up to 50 per cent of total project costs for a total of four years. Consequently, matched funding was set aside from the Foundation's core income for the same time period. The fact that we had access to this kind of core income, rather than having to seek it from external sources, meant that the project did not experience any serious cash-flow difficulties as did some of the other projects in the European Programme.

The total cost for the four years of the project was approximately £160,000, to which the European Commission contributed half. On the Foundation's part, much of the contribution from the core income was used to pay the salary costs of the development officer, with additional project staff being appointed out of the European money. Other major areas of project expenditure included the shop rental and refurbishment, volunteer training and expenses, costs to run CareLine, advertising, administration (including materials such as stationery and printing costs), the production of publicity leaflets, information and materials, and general running costs (heating, lighting, maintenance) associated with any such development. We were also able, as has been indicated above, to obtain other small amounts of funding for quite specific pieces of work associated with the project as it progressed. This included grants obtained under the Department of Health's Opportunities for Volunteering Programme, funds from the Centre for Health and Retirement Education, and Telethon monies.

The long-established policy of the Foundation has been to pilot projects through their initial stages, and then to eventually withdraw when others take on the funding or the project becomes self-financing and independent. In the case of the Self Health Care in Old Age Project, it was felt that by the end of the main funding period (November 1989), there were avenues which the Foundation wished to develop still further (in particular, the advocacy role of peer health counselling). In addition, our close involvement with the local health authority over the initiation and establishment of the project meant that they were willing to explore possible ways of providing more permanent, longer term funding. The outcome of this was that the Elderly Care Unit of the North Staffordshire District Health Authority agreed to co-fund the project until 31 March 1991, with the other 50 per cent being agreed by the Foundation's council and contributed again from its core income.

At about the same time as the health authority agreed to co-fund the project, the Foundation was also successful in obtaining funds from the Opportunities for Volunteering Programme to develop its Peer Health Counselling scheme into an advocacy project. Two years' funding for an advocacy project worker, to recruit and help to train and support more counsellors, was secured. The responsibilities of the post holder also included being organizer of the Senior Centre.

Subsequently, in 1991, the North Staffordshire Health Authority agreed to fund the Senior Health Shop for a further period of 12 months, with a firmly based hope that joint finance funding would be available after this period. The rest of the project's work was absorbed into the Foundation's mainstream expenditure and financed from the core income. In 1992, joint finance funding was awarded for the maximum seven-year period, with the health authority expected to take over the funding at the end of this time. This assured the existence of the project to the turn of the century.

The people

As has become evident, the project was built upon developmental work with older people, by a core group of staff who had been Foundation employees for a number of years. Thus, although the European Poverty Programme money enabled us to get the project up and running, it provided funds to cover only the salaries of certain project staff. In addition as the project, and indeed the Foundation, continued to evolve, this brought with it inevitable changes in terms of staffing.

Neither the Foundation's director, nor the research officer were funded directly under the project and their crucial involvement was undertaken entirely at the Foundation's own expense. This meant that they had other roles and responsibilities over the four years and were therefore not employed full time on the project itself. The Foundation's principal officer (development) was also involved in developments beyond the project itself.

In addition, the project drew on support from administrative staff located at the Foundation's headquarters in Stoke-on-Trent. The Foundation also had a history of supervising social work and nursing students on training placements, which continued over the duration of the project. Social work students helped in the establishment of CareLine (in 1986); observed and participated in the LAY course and in peer health counselling work in residential homes for older people (in 1987); and learnt first hand about how to run recall and physical activity groups in residential homes (in 1988). The shop and the Senior Centre also provided short-term training placements for student nurses from the local hospitals. Last, but by no means least, were the numerous volunteers who worked with us on the project, and whose contributions are assessed in greater detail in Chapter 9.

Local, national and international aspects

Beyond the immediate day-to-day management of the project, there were also a variety of local, national and international networks to which the project related. Specifically, and at a local level, the Foundation itself was managed by a council which itself had two subcommittees, one concerned with projects and one with finance. Members of the council, together with other interested people locally, constituted an advisory group who were able to offer valuable support and advice to staff. Links with the local health authority, with our Members of Parliament and Members of the European Parliament were also important to the development and functioning of the project.

Furthermore, as part of the European Second Poverty Programme, we were also involved in a whole range of activities concerned with cross-national exchange of information, and with a European-wide evaluation process. In the event, a total of 65 action-research projects were funded from the end of 1985. A further 26 projects joined the programme in the summer of 1987 after Spain and Portugal were accepted into the European Community. Out of the 65 original projects, nine were concerned with elderly people. These included two in England (our own, and a mobile bus/drop-in information centre covering part of the rural development area of Lancashire and run by Age Concern Lancashire); two in Wales (a hospital discharge scheme based in Cardiff, and a housing repair scheme run by the Wales Council for Voluntary Action in the Welsh valleys); two in Italy (both based in Rome – one providing help and assistance towards 'extra-care' housing for older people, and the other addressing welfare rights and benefits); one in Luxembourg (being the first day centre to be established in that country); one in France (addressing the needs of elderly male agricultural and craft workers in the rural area of Poitou-Charentes); and one in the Netherlands (a skills-exchange project in Amsterdam).

The Institute Sozialforschung und Gesellschaftspolitik (ISG) in Cologne (Germany), was engaged by the European Commission to develop what was entitled an Animation and Dissemination Service for the entire programme. This service was intended to operate as a clearing house and was responsible for three main tasks:

- *coordination*: promoting continuous collaboration and exchange of information and experience across projects working on the same theme;
- *evaluation*: continuous monitoring of projects and assessment of their significance;
- *dissemination*: publicizing and distributing the results of the programme throughout the European Union.

In order to achieve these aims, the Animation and Dissemination Service appointed two teams of experts: a team of coordinators and a team of evaluators. The coordinators were each responsible for one of the eight themes in the programme. We were therefore required to work together in a cross-national group through the duration of the programme. This involved visits by coordinators to individual projects; meetings of all the projects once or twice a year to exchange experiences and review progress; and occasional exchange activities between project staff and participants.

The evaluation of the whole programme was under the responsibility of the Centre for the Analysis of Social Policy (CASP), Bath University, England. Evaluation activities were organized on a geographical basis (as opposed to themes), and we were assigned an evaluator from the Institute of Local Government Studies at Birmingham University. Evaluation was expected to occur at three levels: by each project monitoring its own activities; through external evaluation by a member of the CASP-appointed team; and at the level of the programme as a whole. Details of our internal evaluation are given in Chapter 6 but, essentially, the external evaluation of our project involved responding to periodic questionnaires, initially to establish a baseline description, and followed subsequently by updating tasks; participation in a two-day working seminar on monitoring and evaluation of the UK projects held in October 1986; in a never-to-be-repeated conference of UK projects examining policy issues held in December 1987; and in periodic visits to the project by the evaluator to examine arrangements for self-evaluation. The expectation was that, in these various ways, systematic evidence of the achievements of the projects could be amassed.

It is not the purpose of this chapter, nor indeed what follows, to comment on the mechanisms that were established to coordinate and externally evaluate the Second European Poverty Programme of which we were a part. Reports of the overall coordination and evaluation are available elsewhere (Greengross and Batty 1989; Room 1990). However, reference will be made to the interaction between the various levels of monitoring and evaluation where relevant. The main focus of the remaining chapters of the book will therefore be oriented around our own internal evaluation of the Self Health Care in Old Age Project, and it is to the features of this that we now turn our attention.

6

Research in action: evaluating the Self Health Care in Old Age Project

Introduction

As we have seen, the Self Health Care in Old Age Project brought together the developmental strands of the Foundation's work into one comprehensive, overarching project. Similarly, it has always been the Foundation's avowed intention to monitor the developments it sets up. The Foundation has a strong commitment to research, believing it to be a worthwhile undertaking and one which is integral to the evolution of a project. The guarantee of four years of co-funding provided us with the first substantial opportunity to integrate fully both the 'action' and the 'research' elements of our work. It is therefore the purpose of this chapter to provide details of the ways in which we went about developing the research aspects of the project. In order to set the particular orientation of this research in context, the chapter will begin with a brief review of the origins of action research. It will then show how and why such an approach seemed to us to be the most appropriate way of monitoring and evaluating our developments. This will be followed by a consideration of what we actually did in our attempt to integrate research and action.

Action research: a review of its development

Action research, as a recognized method of enquiry, dates back at least half a century although its precise origins have been disputed. Kurt Lewin, one of the leading characters in the development of social psychology, is often regarded as an influential force in its evolution, if not the actual founder of action research. Lewin (1946) proposed a model of research which conceived of it as proceeding in a spiral of steps, each of which involved a cycle of planning, action and monitoring (or fact-finding as he termed it). Despite the critiques of Lewin's work and approach over the intervening years (see, for example, Carr and Kemmis 1986; McKernan 1989), his ideas are still a persistent influence on present-day researchers who espouse the value of closer links between practice and research. Not surprisingly, the parameters of what constitutes action research have undergone a great deal of modification and transformation since Lewin's original formulation.

From its initial application in the field of industrial psychology in North America, it spread to Britain both during, and just after, the Second World War. In the field of community affairs, Hart and Bond (1995) trace its development here through the work of the Tavistock Institute and the London School of Economics, and thence to the Community Development Projects (CDPs) spanning the late 1960s to the late 1970s. The CDPs operated in twelve areas of Britain, with the explicit aim of tackling deprivation and poverty through community development work at a grassroots level. Teams of researchers were charged with generating research-based information on which action teams would then base their work. In the true spirit of an action research cycle, these actions were in turn monitored, and the results fed back to the government and the local authority sponsors.

In the educational arena too, the action research paradigm was very influential, particularly in North America, through the work of Corey (1953). After suffering a backlash and decline in interest, it has then been more recently rediscovered in the context of the growing attention being paid to curriculum research and development (McNiff 1988, 1993; McKernan 1991; Nixon 1992). In Britain, since the 1970s, there have been many projects and studies focusing on different aspects of the curriculum, alongside which has come an expansion of networks aimed at supporting the growing numbers of 'practitioner researchers'. Rosemary Webb (1990), in her historical overview of developments in this field, notes too that there have been ideological and methodological splits and disagreements in this movement. Despite this, Hart and Bond (1995: 30) observe that 'critical reflection, grounded in everyday practice, and a problem-focused approach laid the basis for a rediscovery of action research'. Action research has thus become one way of assisting teachers to become more reflexive and critical practitioners.

More recently still, the value of an action research approach has become evident to practitioners and researchers working in contexts other than education. Certainly during the period from the 1980s onwards when we at the Beth Johnson Foundation were beginning to develop the Self Health Care in Old Age Project, there were increasing examples of the employment of action research techniques by people in our own and allied fields, particularly those working in health, social welfare and voluntary sector settings.

In the field of nursing, Christine Webb (1990) and others (Sapsford and Abbott 1992; Holter and Schwartz-Barcott 1993; Sparrow and Robinson 1994) have examined the merits and dimensions involved in this approach. They see it as offering the potential to enhance professional practice, to contribute to organizational and cultural change, and to assist nurses to work with each other, with other professionals and with patients and their families, in ways which might help counter some of the existing power imbalances in these relationships. In similar ways, social work too has had to grapple with trying to inculcate a culture of research-mindedness among practitioners struggling to deal with the day-to-day pressures of the job, and the wider context of seemingly endless reorganization and reforms in the service. As with nursing, commentators on the social work scene, write convincingly about the potential for creating more reflexive practitioners, using action research as the preferred method of choice (Whitaker and Archer 1989; Broad and Fletcher 1993). In the health promotion arena too, where individuals are increasingly encouraged to manage their own health, to develop personal and shared resources for self-care, and to use more formal health services better, a reflexive evaluation approach has very clear parallels with the aims and philosophy of action research (Nutbeam *et al.* 1990; Nutbeam 1998).

Moreover, during the 1980s, the voluntary sector more generally was beginning to advocate the benefits of engaging in self-evaluation alongside developmental work. There was a recognition that a wealth of experience existed among workers and volunteers, which could be enhanced and developed in a research context, in tandem with the work in which people were engaged. With support and guidance it was argued that monitoring and evaluation could, in effect, become an integral part of an organization's day-to-day functioning (Bernard 1992). Fiscal pressures and changes to the funding criteria of voluntary organizations over the 1980s and into the 1990s were also making it increasingly important for such groups to be able to demonstrate the value of what they were doing. Rather than waiting for monitoring and evaluation mechanisms to be imposed from the outside, many groups were keen to develop their own skills and expertise in research, and to be sufficiently informed to decide what was done, who was to do it and to what use it would be put. A flurry of activity in the latter half of the 1980s from organizations such as the Volunteer Centre, and from local voluntary services councils, saw the appearance of a variety of 'how to' guides and related materials (Hedley 1985; Turner and Willis 1987; Ball 1988; Feek 1988; Meadows and Turkie 1988; Birmingham Voluntary Services Council 1989). Arising out of this activity came a demand for local networks and support units such as our own (Bernard *et al.* 1994) and the creation of Charities Evaluation Services, an agency designed to conduct, support and offer training in research and evaluation on a national basis.

In sum then, action research as a means of combining research and action was gaining a substantive foothold during the 1980s in many of the welfare fields allied to our own work in the voluntary sector. At the same time there was, and still is to a great extent, opposition to it from traditional social scientific quarters. As Reinharz (1992: 177) cogently argues, 'contemporary mainstream social science frequently differentiates, rather than integrates, knowledge and action'. Moreover, proponents of the scientific, positivist tradition of social research, tend to regard action research as somehow not 'real research' (Banister *et al.* 1994). This stance though is increasingly being challenged by those who regard a positivist approach to research with people as inappropriate. Work within a qualitative perspective (Lincoln and Guba 1985; Denzin and Lincoln 1994; Gubrium and Sankar 1994; Strauss and Corbin 1998), from those committed to feminist approaches to research (Harding

1986, 1987; Stanley 1990; Reinharz 1992) and within what has been described as 'new paradigm' research (Reason and Rowan 1981; Reason 1988, 1994) are all contributing to a continuing critique of orthodox scientific methods. The tenets of action research as it has evolved in recent years, fit most easily within this broader humanistic approach to social inquiry.

Why choose action research?

In our proposal for European Poverty Programme funding we argued, in line with the World Health Organization (1984), that the promotion of self health care was so underdeveloped that it had not yet been able to generate a corpus of tried and tested research methods, nor was it able to specify what might constitute a successful project. Consequently, researching such a project would itself be breaking new ground. The research was therefore conceived primarily as a means of helping us to constantly review whether the project was meeting its aims and objectives, and to help us decide whether we should change or modify certain aspects as we progressed. It was also our belief that by designing simple and effective research tools, this would contribute to the learning experiences of both participants and staff involved with the project.

Such a rationale suggested to us that an action research cycle was the most appropriate approach to the needs of our project. It will also be remembered from Chapter 5 that one of the conditions of receiving European funding was that projects should have monitoring and evaluation built into them. Our notion of action research as a process of self-monitoring and self-evaluation seemed to fit well with this requirement. Moreover, from the perspective of the development of self health care itself, there were the beginnings in North American writings of this time, of a movement away from research strategies which simply mimicked conventional health education evaluation. Sole reliance on outcome measures such as changes in knowledge, attitudes, behaviour and physiology was increasingly seen as insufficient and inappropriate. These measures were based on the assumption that a simple dose of education could change people's behaviour for the better (Silten and Levin 1979), without any attention being paid to the social, economic, environmental or political contexts within which this 'education' was carried out.

As our own project began to develop we were able to draw on these various strands of existing writing about the value of action research, and clarify more precisely just why we felt that such an approach was suitable. Our own experience in other contexts had long convinced us that there were many reasons why it was important for organizations and groups such as our own to engage in locally based monitoring (Ball and Bernard 1987). Five reasons in particular stood out to us at this time:

- to have an historical record, which can be disseminated to others who may be interested;
- to provide some baseline data to enable us to review how things change over time;
- to enhance, develop and improve our practice or the services we offer;
- to help us make decisions about priorities for the future and to decide where we go next;

- to provide ongoing feedback so that we can review progress and make the necessary alterations.

Our choice of an action research approach, together with the methods and tools we decided to adopt, was approved by our external evaluator and formed the subject of a paper given at a seminar on monitoring and evaluation for all the UK projects in the autumn of 1986 (Robbins 1987a). Expert contributors to this seminar also confirmed the value of projects adopting procedures for self-evaluation, and emphasized the importance of developing ways of expressing what was termed the 'quality side of the balance sheet' as well as the quantity side. Externally, evaluation was seen to be important for three main reasons:

- *pragmatically* – as a condition of the grant; as a way of getting the project's viewpoint across; and as a tool of project management;
- *strategically* – as a way of enabling projects to be reflective and to say what they would do next time; and as a means of sharing discoveries with others;
- *affirmatively* – as a means of developing 'politically persuasive arguments'; to demonstrate what has been achieved in order to influence policy makers; to continue project funding; and to introduce changes.

As the projects developed, the European evaluation team expected to be able to identify key issues across the programme which could then be used to inform their evaluation and be fed back to projects. However, at this stage, both the European Poverty Programme requirements, and the initial embryonic state of our own rationale and plans for self-monitoring and self-evaluation, beg the question of what action research actually consists of. It is this fundamental question which we now attempt to address below.

Action research: definitions, principles and approaches

A great deal of confusion exists over what is precisely meant by the notion of action research. Not surprisingly, given the brief historical review above, there is considerable debate in the literature and in the social research community about what constitutes action research. Much of this debate has taken place since the late 1980s, in the years since we ourselves decided to adopt an action research approach within the Self Health Care in Old Age Project. It is useful to try to clarify the terminology and approaches, however, in order to see where the approach we ourselves adopted fits with the wider literature on this issue.

It was argued earlier that the rediscovery of action research is part of the challenge to orthodox positivist approaches to research with human beings. As such, it shares many of the characteristics and values we have come to associate with the broader term 'qualitative research'. McLeod (1994: 76–8) importantly contends that it is now necessary to examine qualitative research for what it is, rather than as has often been the case, for what it is not; in order to do so he identifies a useful set of fifteen 'interlocking themes, strategies and values characteristic of most qualitative research':

1 *Naturalistic inquiry*: studying real-world phenomena in as unobtrusive a manner as possible, with a sense of openness regarding whatever emerges.

2 *Inductive analysis*: allowing conclusions to arise from a process of immersion in the data, rather than imposing categories or theories decided in advance. A willingness on the part of the researcher to 'bracket-off' his or her assumptions about the phenomena being studied.

3 *An image of an active human subject*: research participants are viewed as purposefully involved in co-creating their social worlds, and are similarly engaged as active co-equals in the research process.

4 *Holistic perspective*: emphasis on the reciprocal interrelationships between phenomena, rather than attempting to create explanations solely in terms of cause–effect sequences. Keeping the larger picture in mind, rather than reducing experience to discrete variables.

5 *Qualitative data*: gathering mainly linguistically based data that are richly descriptive of the experience of informants. Data as 'text' rather than arrays of numbers.

6 *Cyclical nature of research*: any research study involves a cycle of active data-gathering, reflective interpretation and assessment of the accuracy of findings.

7 *Personal contact and insight*: the researcher is in close contact with the people being studied. The quality of the researcher–informant relationship is of critical importance. The use of the researcher's empathic understanding of informants as a source of data.

8 *Process orientation*: views the phenomena being investigated as a dynamic system where change is constant and ongoing.

9 *Awareness of uniqueness*: a willingness to view each individual case as special and unique. The principle of respecting the particular configuration of individual cases even when developing general conclusions.

10 *Contextual awareness*: findings can be understood only within a social, cultural, historical and environmental context. Part of the task of the researcher is to consider these contextual factors.

11 *Design flexibility*: within a study, methods and procedures are adapted in response to new circumstances and experiences.

12 *Flexible sampling*: the choice of participants in a study is determined by a range of theoretical and practical considerations, not merely by the aim of accumulating a 'representative' subset of the general population.

13 *Reflexivity*: the idea that the researcher is his or her primary instrument, and as a result must be aware of the fantasies, expectations and needs that his or her participation introduces to the research process.

14 *Empowerment as a research goal*: an awareness of the social and political implications of research, accompanied by a commitment to using the research process to benefit the participants.

15 *A constructionist approach to knowledge*: taking the point of view that reality is socially constructed (Gergen 1985). The products of research are not 'facts' or 'findings' that reflect an objective reality, but are versions of the life-world that are constructed by the researcher (or co-constructed between researcher and participants).

Action research does not subscribe to every single one of these features, but it does share the fundamental goal of qualitative research which is to 'uncover and illuminate what things mean to people' (McLeod 1994: 78). For us, at least two-thirds of the features identified by McLeod resonate with the approach we adopted in the Self Health Care in Old Age Project.

Our approach aimed to ensure that we incorporated the following elements in our research:

- a cyclical process;
- a holistic and naturalistic perspective;
- an appreciation of the context of our work;
- a process orientation;
- design flexibility and reflexivity;
- awareness of the importance of the quality of the researcher–informant relationship;
- an image of project participants as co-equals in the research process;
- empowerment as a goal of the research as well as the project.

Moreover, as McLeod (1994) notes, some of the features of qualitative research are also present in certain kinds of quantitative studies which is a further reason why we, in our project, decided to incorporate both quantitative and qualitative measures as will be seen below.

Detailing a wide range of characteristic elements in this way provides us with a broad understanding of the constituent parts of action research. However, many writers have attempted to refine these down in order to delineate the essentials of an action research approach. These 'essentials' or 'core characteristics' range from the three distinctive features of intervention, context specificity and the development of theory from findings, identified by Lathlean (1994); to the five forms of 'feminist change-oriented research' delineated by Reinharz (1992: 180); and the seven distinguishing criteria in Hart and Bond's (1995) action research typology.

Reinharz (1992: 180) argues for the centrality of 'change' in all feminist research. She also devotes a chapter of her book to discussing five types of research with what she calls 'an explicit action connection', each of which draws on all the techniques in the social sciences as opposed to just one particular methodological orientation. These five types, with very abbreviated descriptions, are as follows:

- *Action research* – research in which action and evaluation are carried out simultaneously. Such action research projects attempt to directly change people's behaviour. Data about these changes are gathered in either traditional or innovative ways, and the project proceeds in a continuous series of feedback loops.
- *Participatory or collaborative research* – which involves the people being studied in all phases of the research process. Empowerment is a central goal of this kind of research, which aims to create both social and individual change by altering the role relations of those involved in the project.
- *Prevalence and needs assessment* – often reliant on surveys, this kind of research attempts to determine the absolute or relative numbers of people who have a particular need or experience. Such research can have the effect of mobilizing people to respond to the needs or problems which have

been identified, as well as contributing to consciousness raising and preventive activities.

- *Evaluation research* – research with the purpose of evaluating the effectiveness of different types of action in meeting needs or solving problems. It
can be used at both individual and organizational levels, or to evaluate
evaluation research itself. It is frequently employed where people are concerned to improve their own practice and create a blueprint which others
can follow. It should preferably focus not simply on the results of participation in an activity or project, but on the process elements as well.
- *Demystification* – research within this kind of framework subscribes to the
view that the very act of obtaining knowledge creates the potential for
change. Because of the paucity of research on certain groups, this tends to
accentuate and perpetuate their powerlessness and invisibility. Demystification is closely linked to self-education, the sharing of information, consciousness raising, and a desire for people to learn from the experiences of
others.

Again, our own project, and the research orientation that we adopted, have
quite clear philosophical and methodological links with all five types of
change-oriented research identified here.

Finally, it is instructive to examine the Hart and Bond (1995) typology.
Building on their reading of the action research literature, and on their
experiences as action researchers, they distinguish seven criteria as a framework for their typology. Action research:

1 is educative;
2 deals with individuals as members of social groups;
3 is problem-focused, context specific and future-orientated;
4 involves change intervention;
5 aims at improvement and involvement;
6 involves a cyclic process in which research, action and evaluation are
  interlinked;
7 is founded on a research relationship in which those involved are participants in the change process.

(Hart and Bond 1995: 37–8)

These criteria are 'interlinked facets of the action research process, so that in
practice they overlap and interweave' (Hart and Bond 1995: 48). The particular configurations of these parameters will also vary according to the particular type of action research in which they are located. Their four ideal
types, again with brief descriptions, are as follows:

- *Experimental* – closely associated with the early days of action research and
the scientific approach to social problems. It is researcher focused and
researcher managed, using experimental intervention to test and/or generate theory. The research elements tend to dominate, and it is usually time
limited and task focused, with the aim of identifying causal processes that
can be generalized. The researcher is likely to be external and to have a
clearly differentiated role from that of the practitioners.
- *Organizational* – in which action research is applied to organizational

problem solving in order to overcome resistance to change and create more productive working relationships. A managerially biased or client focused, top-down approach aiming at tangible outcomes. Action and research often in tension, with rational sequential process and differentiated roles.

- *Professionalizing* – in which practice informs the research and where the 'new' professions such as teaching, nursing and social work are attempting to develop research-based practice in order to enhance their status in line with the more established professions. Encourages the development of reflective practice and aims to empower professionals to advocate on behalf of their clients/patients. Problems to be investigated emerge from professional practice. Although research and action are in tension, the research tends to dominate and is carried out through a dynamic and opportunistic spiral of cycles. Practitioner and researcher roles merge.
- *Empowering* – most closely associated with community development approaches in which an explicit anti-oppressive stance is taken. Aims to shift the balance of power, raise consciousness and empower oppressed groups. User/practitioner focused in which problems to be addressed are negotiated. A bottom-up, process-led approach which expects and accepts that the research process, explanations and solutions will be fluid, pluralistic and open-ended. Although the action components dominate, roles are negotiated and shared.

This typology can be read and interpreted in various ways. At one level, it represents a historical dimension showing how action research has developed over time from a scientific approach to a more qualitative and social constructionist methodology. Considered as a continuum, it also highlights how the relative weights we might attach to 'action' and 'research' can lead to different kinds of studies. Importantly too, Hart and Bond (1995: 46–7) acknowledge that any given action research project may in fact shift between the different types during its lifetime, perhaps from being outcome led and weighted towards research, to being process led and weighted towards action.

Research in action: the Self Health Care in Old Age Project

From the perspective of the Self Health Care in Old Age Project, it is interesting to observe that the research elements of our first proposal (the one which did not receive funding from the Health Education Council) were largely conceived within the Hart and Bond (1995) experimental type of action research and driven, to a great extent, by the expectations of those we saw as potential funders. In this original proposal, it was anticipated that the project's activities would be monitored and evaluated through quasi-experimental means, alongside an examination of the project's historical development. In particular, the research outline stressed the importance of measurable outcomes for clients, using a before and after design and matching them with a control group who did not come into contact with the project's activities. There was a strong emphasis on objectively measured changes, including things like blood pressure, weight, lung function and resting pulse. A 'health biographies' project was to complement this work, and there would need to be a research team comprising the research officer, a research assistant and a series of internal, specially trained assessors along the lines of the 'Quality of Life' studies carried out in the 1970s (Perry 1977).

This researcher-oriented top-down approach had (as indicated in Chapter 5) to be considerably modified. In effect, this meant that we were able to return to a research framework which was more closely allied to the philosophical and conceptual basis around which the Foundation organized most of its work. Pragmatically too, the available funding from the European Commission did not allow us to create a vast and labour-intensive research structure. As in our past history, we were thrown back on our own internal resources and had to devise ways of making the best possible use of the skills and abilities of those involved with the project, in research as well as in developmental terms. We were also much more comfortable, individually and as a group, operating towards the empowering end of the Hart and Bond (1995) typology. Both the Foundation's director and the development officer had come from social work/community development backgrounds and had been employed by the Foundation for many years. They also felt confident that I, though academically trained, had gained sufficient experience in my two and a half years with the Foundation to be sensitive to the particular research needs and requirements of a voluntary organization.

Like any research, action research needs to be planned and guided by some kind of framework which conveys a sense of what it is one is interested in finding out. As a consequence, and drawing on the aims and principles of the project as outlined in Chapter 5 together with the self-empowerment factors discussed in Chapter 3, we were able to develop and agree between us a broad and flexible framework for the research. Two main aims of the research were identified:

- To monitor the processes involved in setting up the project, and in developing its various elements over the funding period.
- To evaluate the impact of the project on the self health care activities of older people in North Staffordshire.

We also stressed the importance of the close interlinkage between research and action, and of the involvement of all staff in both aspects: 'It is important that the monitoring and evaluation feeds back into the development of the project and, conversely, that developers become actively engaged in the monitoring and evaluation process' (Creber *et al.* 1985: 4).

Once funding was secured, we subsequently agreed that our own internal monitoring and evaluation strategy would be organized around the following three foci:

- *Process of development* – prior to, and throughout the project's lifetime, detailed records were to be kept. This would enable us to produce a chronology of the project, describing the fine details of how it came about; how finance was secured; what was developed when; and how it was organized and run on a day-to-day basis. Apart from providing an ongoing account of the development of the project, this was considered to be important for others who might wish to learn from what we were doing or borrow elements of it.

- *Quantitative information* – was to be collected in order to provide some 'hard' facts and figures about the people who became involved with the project and its various elements. This would help us to determine, for example, who the project was reaching and what kinds of effects it was having on them.
- *Qualitative information* – was to be used to supplement the process and quantitative aspects. As an innovative project concerned with the quality of life of older people, we felt strongly that more was required than just bare statistics if we were to accurately reflect what was happening to those whom the project touched. The emphasis here was to explore in some depth what the project meant to certain individuals, in the context of their life experiences.

These foci needed then to be translated into actual research techniques and tools. Before describing these, it is interesting to observe that our three foci reflect yet a further way of interpreting the Hart and Bond (1995: 47–8) typology. They indicate that it can be read as treating action research as a technique with the 'experimental' end involving traditional quantitative research designs, and the 'empowering' end involving a more integrated process-led approach. A third position recognizes that 'during the life of a project it may encompass both quantitative and qualitative approaches for which participatory action research forms a framework' (Hart and Bond 1995: 48). Quite clearly, the framework for our project accords very closely with this third position.

Research in action: chosen methods

By its very nature, action research not only draws on diverse disciplines, but also makes use of a whole variety of methods (Reinharz 1992; Banister *et al.* 1994). In the copious literature which now exists on social research methods, such an approach to data generation and analysis may be referred to as multi-method or multiple methods research, as pluralistic evaluation or as triangulation. The underlying assumption of such an approach is that any conclusions one might draw will be all the stronger if there is supporting evidence from a variety of different sources. It also enables findings from one type of study to be checked out against another, and consequently allows for the possibility that convergent data may not be produced (Bryman 1992). Rather, competing and differing interpretations of the same events and materials may need to be discussed. In the end though, the hope is that a more thorough and complete understanding of critical issues might emerge (Reinharz 1992; McLeod 1994).

Since the mid-1980s, the research literature has become replete with arguments and debates about whether, and how, true methodological pluralism can ever be achieved (Bryman 1988; Brannen 1992). However, from the perspective of our own project, it was patently obvious that whatever difficulties we might encounter in carrying out a multi-method approach, reliance on a single type of data or method of analysis would be doomed to failure before it started. The only way of attempting to do justice to an innovative and many-faceted project had to lie with research that attempted to capture some of this dynamism and complexity.

Table 6.1 Monitoring and evaluation tools employed for each project activity

	Senior Health Shop	Peer health counselling	CareLine	Health-related activities
Process	Documentation. Minutes. Action plans. Photographs. Publicity. Visitor records. Presentations. Enquiry sheets.	Documentation. Minutes (monthly support group meetings). Action plans. Photographs. Publicity. Visitor records. Presentations. Enquiry sheets.	Documentation. Minutes (monthly support group meetings). Action plans. Photographs. Publicity. Visitor records. Presentations. Enquiry sheets.	Documentation. Minutes. Action plans. Photographs. Publicity. Visitor records. Presentations. Enquiry sheets.
Quantitative information	Quarterly census weeks (questionnaire interviews; counts; observation). Bi-annual census weeks (self-completion questionnaires). Short response forms. Computer response forms. Daily diary. Enquiry book. Attendance records. Leaflet and resource material counts.	Pre and post-training questionnaires (participants and staff). Course/training attendance records. Session response forms. Weekly report forms. Peer health counselling logs.	Pre and post-training questionnaires (participants and staff). Course/training attendance records. Training feedback forms. Referral sheets. Assessment forms. Client information files.	Attendance registers. Feedback forms. Self-monitoring forms.
Qualitative information	Participant observation. Non-participant observation. Field notes. Interviews (staff, volunteers, participants). Photographs.	Peer health counselling logs. Shadowing. Case reviews. Testimonials/letters. Interviews (staff, volunteers, participants). Photographs.	Participant observation (of training). Video recording (of training). Case reviews. Non-participant observation. Testimonials/letters. Interviews (staff, volunteers, participants). Photographs.	Participant observation. Non-participant observation. Interviews (staff, volunteers, participants). Photographs. 'Open response' paragraphs.

In order to do so, it was recognized that different methods of data collection would be appropriate with the different elements which went to make up the project, and at different points during the lifetime of the project. Our proposal had argued the case that while the research could obviously utilize some existing tools and methodologies, it also needed 'to develop other robust, and perhaps less "scientific" strategies and indicators in order to encourage constructive feedback into the development of the project' (Creber *et al.* 1985: 3). At the formative stage of the development of the proposal, it was both inappropriate and exceedingly difficult to specify precisely in what combination, or order, we might use particular methods or tools. Much of this was dependent on the ways in which the elements which went to make up the project were developed. We were aware, though, that we would need to draw on a whole range of both conventional, and perhaps not-so-conventional techniques.

Beattie (1991) has subsequently coined the term 'portfolio approach', which seems an apt description for what we were trying to do. He defines six broad categories which have since been adapted and modified by Hart and Bond (1995: 206):

- *Basic work records* – attendance, costs, diaries, logs, minutes, memos, workplans, activity profiles.
- *Needs database* – local health statistics, local survey findings, practice reports, interviews.
- *Project file* – time charts, curriculum vitae of project workers, job descriptions, agendas and minutes of meetings, research diaries and activity logs.
- *Audits* – summaries of feedback sessions from users/clients, consumer satisfaction surveys, letters of complaint and/or thanks, evaluation and free comment sheets.
- *Follow-up data* – learning contracts, action plans, pledges/pleas, digests of follow-up surveys.
- *External monitor* – press cuttings, testimonials, conference presentations, publications.

In their discussion of action research, Banister *et al.* (1994: 114–15) not only affirm these methods of data collection, but also advise action researchers of the additional need to consider

- *Observation and shadowing.*
- *Tape/video recording and still photographs.*

In sum, we wanted to monitor and evaluate the individual elements of the project as well as trying to gain an understanding of the project as a whole. We expected to have to use an array of research tools, and Table 6.1 attempts to convey the variety of instruments we employed in order to assess the project's development. The four main activities of the project are listed across the top of the table, with the three foci for the research down the left-hand side. In each cell of the table are indicated, from the above portfolio of techniques, which tools were used to monitor and evaluate each activity. When examining the table, the reader should bear in mind that this is a simplified summary of what we did. It is not meant to imply that all these methods were used all the time, throughout the duration of the project!

Dissemination activities

For the information and experience gained through the project to be of any use to others, it is also vital that dissemination procedures are incorporated as an integral part of the overall research design: internal and external dissemination are equally important, and overlapping. Internally, the Foundation produced (and still does) a monthly newsletter for all the groups and organizations under its umbrella. This gave up-to-date information about events and activities, including the Self Health Care in Old Age Project. In addition, minutes of the regular review meetings and ensuing action plans (detailed in Table 6.1) were widely circulated within the project.

In terms of external dissemination, we adopted a number of techniques as detailed below:

- *Project newsletter* – twelve issues of *UPDATE* (the bulletin of the North Staffordshire Self Health Care in Old Age Project) were compiled during the initial period of project funding, with a final two issues appearing in summer 1990 and winter 1991. Edited by the research officer, and subsequently by the director, the newsletter was used to publicize and inform people about the progress of the project. It was mailed out to people in the UK and abroad, thus ensuring a wide readership for those interested in this aspect of the Foundation's work.
- *Information packs and leaflets* – a whole variety of leaflets were produced during the project's lifetime which gave people information about the various activities being undertaken. These were free on request.
- *Reports and other writings* – short reports on different elements of the project were produced by various staff members and students who worked with us. Half way through the period of project funding, an interim report was produced and, in January 1990, the director compiled a 'final' report to the European Commission. During and indeed since the initial period of project funding, the core staff (both individually and collaboratively) have also contributed articles to popular and academic journals.
- *Presentations* – project staff have all been involved in presenting the project to local, national and international seminars and conferences, as well as to groups of older people and professionals who work with them. For example, presentations have been made at social clubs, on qualifying training courses for health and social work students, at in-service training sessions, and on pre-retirement courses.
- *Media coverage* – the Foundation was fortunate in having good contacts with both local radio and the local press. News items about the project appeared regularly in these media with, on one occasion, a local radio presenter doing his entire morning programme from the Senior Health Shop. The project has featured on national radio, in various magazine articles, as part of the Age Well information packs (HEC/Age Concern England 1985; HEA/Age Concern England 1988) and in several television programmes aimed at older people (such as in one of Central Television's *Getting On* programmes in early 1988).
- *Visit Days* – it was noted in Chapter 5 that after the first nine months of the project, we felt it necessary to introduce monthly Visit Days which continued

for the rest of the initial funding period. Groups of visitors (usually between four and ten) have come from all over the UK and from abroad, and have been able to see and hear first hand about our developments. In addition, 'special' visitor days have been arranged for larger groups of staff and/or students from, for example, the health authority, the Social Services Department, housing associations and nearby Keele University. In April 1988, the Senior Health Shop was visited by Mrs Edwina Currie, then a Minister of Health in the Conservative government.

Assessing the impact of such dissemination activities is very difficult although we are aware that at least some of our visitors have taken up certain of the ideas and activities they have seen for use in their own areas.

Conclusion

The preceding pages have attempted to trace the influences on our own action research project and to provide the reader with some sense of what we actually did during the first four years of project funding. What we hope has become clear is that action research of the kind we were engaged in is not a value-free undertaking. It takes place within a social and political context and has to take account of both wider societal influences and local pressures. This will, almost inevitably, create tensions at various levels within the project and over time. However, an action research approach which involved us as staff, together with volunteers and the older people who came into contact with the project, seemed to us the most appropriate way of trying to address these issues.

The eventual action research design in fact brought together half a dozen disparate strands and influences. First, it closely reflected the philosophy of the organization itself (the Beth Johnson Foundation) which had developed a policy of working 'with', as opposed to 'for', older people in creative and innovative ways. Second, research on the development of self health care activities in Britain was very poorly developed, and appeared to us to illustrate the need for descriptive monitoring and close examination of any new initiative. Third, our own professional histories, and indeed personal inclinations, were also an influence on the ways in which we chose to work. With backgrounds in community development work and social research, we preferred to operate in as participatory and collaborative a fashion as possible, trying to retain the needs of our target group – older people – at the forefront of whatever we did. Fourth, the nature of the funding available from the European Commission meant that we had to demonstrate clearly in the proposal, the means by which we would monitor and evaluate our own developments. Fifth, the project was part of the much wider European Second Poverty Programme, which itself was keen to build on the lessons from the first programme and from the earlier American Anti-Poverty Program and the British Community Development Projects. Finally, our external evaluator had himself been closely involved with the British CDPs, and was very supportive of what we were trying to achieve. Action research as a strategy offered us the means of combining all these strands together in ways which we hoped would be truly empowering for all of us involved with the project. The next three chapters will move beyond the details of what we did, to consider the impact which the project had on older people, volunteers and staff.

7

Self health care in action: participation, accessibility and informed choice among older people

Introduction

We have seen in previous chapters that the project was organized around a number of broad aims, and was directed towards trying to articulate the model of self-empowered health behaviour outlined at the close of Chapter 3. The dimensions of this model, together with the professed aims of the project, suggested to us that there were a number of internal, project-generated criteria against which it might be possible to assess the impact of the scheme. First, our overriding aim was to encourage the participation of older people in a variety of health-related activities. *Participation* was therefore one of the main criteria with which we were concerned.

On the surface, participation is about numbers: how many people came through the doors of the Senior Health Shop and of the Senior Centre; how many people engage in the variety of activities on offer, and so on. Behind the numbers, however, it was important to us to learn more about who these people were, what factors facilitated or constrained their ability to participate, and how they felt about their participation at whatever level. Consequently, participation is intimately bound up with the following crucial criteria:

- *Accessibility* – of the various elements of the project, including physical access, access to written information, and access to a variety of professional and para-professional support and advice.
- *Informed choice* – the extent to which people have the information they need and want in order to be able to make real choices about the options which may be open to them.
- *Skills development* – which encompasses the acquisition of identifiable,

practical skills as well as the development of confidence, self-esteem and self-identity.

If the project was successful in providing these opportunities, then it was our hope that the older people who chose to become involved would feel a very real sense, finally, of:

- *Empowerment* – through the raising of awareness, knowledge, understanding and competence.

In addition, the European evaluation team selected three criteria which they felt would be useful for assessing the achievements of all the projects under the Second Poverty Programme (Room 1990). The three European criteria were as follows:

- *Participation* – the extent to which the project has been designed and implemented with the participation of the target group itself.
- *Cost effectiveness* – to include both readily observed and easily costed inputs and outputs, as well as the often concealed non-resource based inputs and outputs.
- *Innovation* – what parallel or new perspectives are drawn upon to contribute to the development of useful knowledge and methods; and to address deficiencies and gaps in existing policy and practice.

These seven criteria – *participation, accessibility, informed choice, skills development, empowerment, cost effectiveness and innovation* – are used to organize discussion about the impact which the project had on older people, volunteers and staff. Given that the focus of this book is on self-evaluation, the two external European criteria relating to cost effectiveness and innovation are not addressed here. While we certainly wished to make the best use of our resources (although we, like other projects, were anxious that this should not be equated with 'cheapness') and believed that our project was innovative, judgements about this are, and indeed were, more appropriately made by our external evaluators (Greengross and Batty 1989; Room 1990). Furthermore, rather than attempting to distil data from the entire array of monitoring and evaluation techniques employed (see Table 6.1), the present discussions draw selectively from the work which was carried out in order to illustrate specific points.

This chapter therefore concentrates on older people themselves, and focuses on the first three criteria of participation, accessibility and informed choice. It details some of the hard facts and figures (our quantitative data), before moving on to look at more qualitative aspects in subsequent sections. These discussions are illustrated with particular reference to the Senior Health Shop. The focus of Chapter 8 will then be on the older people who participated in various health-related activities (notably the Look After Yourself courses), looking in particular at the criteria of skills development and empowerment. Discussion of the impact on volunteers and staff forms the subject of Chapter 9 and concentrates on the work of peer health counsellors and CareLine.

However, it is important for the reader to bear in mind that these distinctions are somewhat artificial. Older people were of course participants in all four elements of the project. Likewise, the volunteers were mostly older people themselves, and were able to move flexibly around the project perhaps being a participant in one area of activity, but a volunteer in another. Similarly staff, while retaining overall responsibility for the project, were also able at times to become active participants.

In essence then, both this and the succeeding chapters attempt to address three basic questions:

* Who became involved with the project?
* What kinds of health-related activities did they engage in?
* What impact did their participation have on them?

Given that the shop was literally the shop window for other aspects of the project, then Senior Health Shop records provide the main source of information for this chapter. In this instance, much of the information is presented in descriptive rather than in tabular form. Readers interested in the detailed statistics are encouraged to refer to other articles and chapters about the project which have appeared since the mid-1980s (see, for example, Creber *et al.* 1985; Ivers 1985; Bernard and Ivers 1986; Bernard 1988, 1989, 1993, 1998).

Participation at the Senior Health Shop

The absence of the research officer on maternity leave at the time of the shop opening (in August 1986) meant that systematic recording of attendance did not begin until October of that year. Over the initial period of project funding, attendance at the shop increased steadily. During the first full calendar year of operation, there were 5500 attendances. In the following two years, this figure doubled to approximately 11,000 per year. Attendance then settled down to between 800 and 1000 people per month meaning that, on average, between 40 and 50 people come to the shop each day.

These average figures mask daily and weekly fluctuations, and give no indication of the ways in which attendance responds to things like the weather conditions or publicity for the project. An examination of the daily diary and weekly reports for 1988 provides an illustration of these points. On 15 January, a feature article about the project appeared in the local paper, the *Evening Sentinel*. The next day, 34 people came in directly as a result of having read about it. The weekly report recalls how the shop was 'buzzing with conversations' all that day. For the next fortnight too, attendances were up (from 185 in the week of the article, to 249 the following week and 282 the week after that) with many people indicating that the article had prompted them to come and have a look. We can track similar patterns of increased attendance in response to monthly broadcasts made by the development officer on the local radio station; to the reported visit to the shop by Mrs Edwina Currie on 7 April 1988; to an article which appeared in a national magazine in May; and to a Radio 4 broadcast about the project in early September.

Who came?

Attendance figures obviously give us an overall impression of numbers. However, we (and our external evaluators) were also interested in who these people coming through the doors were. Two principal means were employed to gather this kind of information (see Table 6.1). First, at each table in the shop there were very short response forms which took about five minutes for customers to fill in by themselves. This form sought brief socio-demographic data; asked customers how they knew about the shop; and explored what they had done while visiting, as well as what they intended to do. Completed forms would then be posted in a box at the reception desk on the way out.

Second, we also carried out what we termed quarterly 'census weeks'. In the first full year, these census weeks consisted of a total count of everyone who came into the shop; face-to-face questionnaire interviews with every second customer; and observations of the general day-to-day running and interactions which took place. (These continued in a modified self-completion format after the research officer moved in 1988 to take up an appointment at the nearby university, and have subsequently been conducted bi-annually since 1989.) The interviews made use of a simple four-page questionnaire which asked for social and personal information about customers; how they had heard about the shop; why they had come; what aspects of health they were particularly interested in; and what they planned to do, or had already done, to improve their own health and well-being. Their opinions of the shop, and their views about what other kinds of services, advice or health-related groups might be of interest to them, were also sought.

Together, the census weeks and the short response forms provide us with a range of socio-demographic data about participants at the shop. These data are presented here in the form of simple descriptive statistics, due primarily to the fact that the Foundation's resources meant that all analysis of monitoring and evaluation material had to be undertaken manually.

Over the initial funding period, a total of ten census weeks were held (quarterly in 1987 and 1988, and twice in 1989). During this time, 829 people over the age of 50 were interviewed or self-completed the questionnaire (after the change in 1988). Of these 814 indicated their sex (the change to a self-completion format meant inevitably that there were a number of instances of missing data), of whom 648 (80 per cent) were women and 166 (20 per cent) were men. In other words, female shop customers outnumbered their male counterparts by four to one, although there were slight variations in these proportions at different censuses.

Data from the short response forms confirm this general pattern. It was possible to determine the sex of the respondent on 414 of these forms (out of a total of 454 which were returned), of whom 300 (72 per cent) were women and 114 (28 per cent) were men. This indicates that men perhaps preferred the greater anonymity afforded by this method of monitoring, since the ratio of women to men is somewhat lower than the average for the census weeks.

In terms of age, by far the greatest proportion of participants are people in their sixties: over half of respondents each year are in this age group. A fifth of customers are in their fifties and the same proportion are in their seventies. Only very small minorities of people are aged 80 or over, although the age of customers has ranged from 50 to 87 years.

Perhaps unsurprisingly, when we look at the data for age and sex combined, we find that male customers tend to be overwhelmingly in their sixties.

At the December census in 1988 for example, 70 per cent of the men were in this age range. The age distribution for women is much wider, reflecting both the fact that at the 'younger' end of the age range the shop attracted substantial numbers of women in their fifties and also that women, as we know, generally outlive men. So, we discover a consistent pattern in the data with approximately 20 per cent of women customers being in their fifties, 50 per cent in their sixties, 25 per cent in their seventies and a small minority in their eighties. Moreover, the ratios of women to men are highest for those customers in their fifties, and in their seventies and beyond. In the group of customers in their fifties, women have outnumbered men at the different censuses in ratios of between four to one and eight to one; while at seventy and above the ratio has been as high as twelve to one.

These gender imbalances are further reflected in the other sociodemographic information we have. On average, over one-half of the respondents are married and one-third or more are widowed. Half of respondents live with their spouse, and between one-third and two-fifths live alone. However, in keeping with broader demographic trends, it is the women rather than the men who tend to be both widowed and living alone, particularly as they move into their seventies and eighties (at some censuses, 80 per cent of women this age were in this situation). Men, by contrast, tend to be married and living with their spouse.

To supplement this profile of participants, we collected data relating to people's housing, what their levels of income were and how they rated their own health. Averaged out over the ten censuses (total sample = 829 people), 60 per cent of people owned their homes outright, with a further 12 per cent still buying on a mortgage. Older people have shared in the general growth of home ownership and this sample was no exception. A further 17 per cent of respondents rented from the local council, while 5 per cent rented privately (the remaining 6 per cent were divided between other forms of tenure or declined to disclose this information). In terms of the kinds of housing in which people lived, it is important to observe that the Potteries is an area with a legacy of Victorian terraced housing, particularly around the centres of the six main towns (Hanley, Burslem, Tunstall, Stoke, Longton and Fenton). Thus, although two-fifths (42 per cent) of the sample lived in semi-detached houses, nearly a quarter (23 per cent) still lived in terraced houses. A further fifth (19 per cent) lived in bungalows, with small minorities of respondents living in detached houses (8 per cent), flats (6 per cent) or sheltered accommodation (1 per cent).

We were also able to gather information, albeit crudely, about people's levels of income. This was important given the fact that the project was part of the European Poverty Programme – although it will be remembered that our definition of poverty was one that encompassed dimensions other than just monetary ones. Thus, the questionnaire asked people to indicate in broad terms what the level of their household's total weekly income was, and how many people contributed to this total. For those people who were living in households consisting of more than one person, this obviously gives us no indication of the way in which household income was distributed between individuals. It did though allow us to make some basic calculations. Furthermore, it is important to observe here that income, perhaps more so than any other topic, is an issue which people are very circumspect about discussing. Our respondents were no exception and, on average, one in six people (17 per cent or 141 people) over the ten censuses declined to answer this question. Out of a total of 829 respondents, we therefore have information concerning the incomes of 688 people.

Bearing in mind these cautions, our data show that about half (49 per cent) of people who responded were at that time managing on an income of less than £50 per week, in essence, the basic state pension. A further third (33 per cent) had between £50 and £100 per week; one-tenth (12 per cent) between £100 and £200; and a tiny minority (2 per cent) in excess of £200. A small proportion (4 per cent) of respondents did not know what their income was. What this reveals is that considerable numbers of older people being reached by the project were living on very low incomes indeed. Again, women tended to predominate among those in the lowest two income categories.

Finally, we asked people to rate their health on a scale from excellent to very poor as shown in Table 7.1.

As can be seen, there are no very great differences between the sexes, although slightly higher proportions of men rate their health as either excellent or good, while higher proportions of women rate their health as fair. Comparison with larger scale sample surveys such as the General Household Survey (GHS: see OPCS 1993) and the Health and Lifestyles Survey (HALS: see Cox *et al.* 1987) suggests that both the men and women in our sample tend to rate their health rather more favourably. Sidell (1995) shows, for example, that 45 per cent of women in the HALS survey, and 38 per cent in the GHS assess their health as good, compared with 60 per cent of our female respondents. Likewise, 44 per cent of men in both the HALS and GHS samples rate their health as good in comparison with 66 per cent of our respondents.

Explanations for these differences may, however, be as much to do with different ways of rating as with any 'real' differences between the samples. Our study employed a five-point scale, the HALS a four-point scale and the GHS a three-point scale, which may be a contributory factor in the more favourable assessments of their health held by our respondents. Additionally, our respondents are aged 50 and above, while the other two surveys deal with people over the age of 65 who, arguably, may be less likely to be so optimistic.

Table 7.1   Senior Health Shop respondents: women's and men's health status

	Excellent		Good		Fair		Poor/very poor		Total
	n	*(%)*	*n*	*(%)*	*n*	*(%)*	*n*	*(%)*	*n*
1987 Women	10	(6)	92	(58)	52	(33)	4	(3)	158
Men	2	(5)	26	(67)	8	(21)	3	(8)	39
1988 Women	22	(7)	190	(61)	92	(30)	7	(2)	311
Men	11	(12)	57	(63)	18	(20)	4	(4)	90
1989 Women	11	(7)	103	(62)	48	(29)	5	(3)	167
Men	3	(9)	23	(68)	7	(21)	1	(3)	34

A more direct comparison can be made with the British Gas Attitudes to Ageing survey, which showed that 78 per cent of interviewees reported themselves as in 'very good' or 'fairly good' health (Midwinter 1991: 15). Nonetheless, it is important to remind ourselves again here that a positive, but subjective, assessment of one's health does not preclude the possibility that one might also be 'objectively' unwell at the same time (see Chapter 1).

Discussion: reaching out to people

Taken together, this social and demographic information shows that the shop custom was clearly dominated by older women. Those women in their fifties were usually married and living with their spouse, and had household incomes somewhat above the basic state pension. Those aged 70 and over tended to be widowed, living alone and were surviving on less than £50 per week. These findings are important in that they reveal that our project was reaching sections of the older female population whom research at that time was beginning to show tended, for a variety of reasons, to be 'missed' or poorly served by formal health services. Ford and Taylor (1985), for example, argue that 'middle-aged' women – defined as being aged 45–64 – are one of the groups who run the greatest risk of neglecting their own health problems. In addition, the work on informal carers, which also gathered pace during the 1980s, revealed that this self-same group of women were the ones most likely to be caring for other family members (Green 1988). One possible consequence of this was that their overriding concern for their dependants would, once again, lead to them ignoring their own health needs. For some other older women, including those of our customers in their seventies and beyond, there are indications that older people are dissatisfied with certain aspects of health care services (Wenger 1988; Sidell 1993, 1995). We therefore thought that it was possible that women might be coming to the shop precisely because they were experiencing similar concerns. This observation leads us naturally to a consideration of how accessible the shop was, what customers came to do there, and how they felt about what they found.

Accessibility of the Senior Health Shop

By siting the shop in Hanley, the commercial centre, it was hoped to draw participants from across the Potteries as well as from North Staffordshire. This has indeed proved to be the case. Just over one-quarter of customers come from within a radius of one mile: from Hanley itself and from areas in the immediate vicinity which ring the town centre. A further quarter travel in from between one and two miles away and another quarter or more come from between two and four miles away. In other words, three-quarters of the people who come to the shop live within the Potteries, many travelling in by bus to the main bus station, a five-minute walk away. Of the remainder, 15 per cent travel in from towns adjacent to the main urban area, while approximately 5 per cent come from further afield. This is to say nothing of customers who come from far greater distances (or indeed overseas), who have usually been visiting relatives in the area and have been brought in to 'have a look'.

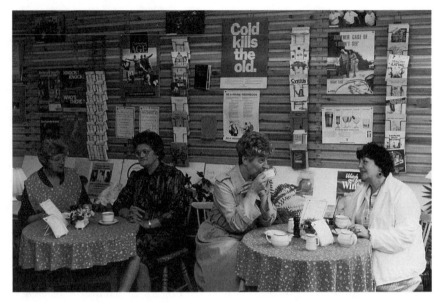

The interior of the Senior Health Shop

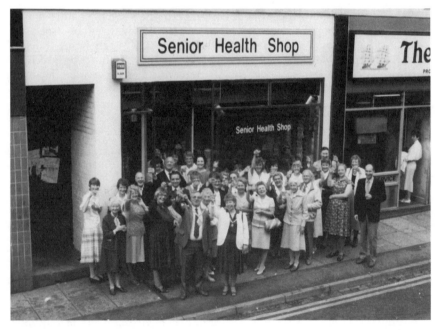

The Senior Health Shop celebrates its first year

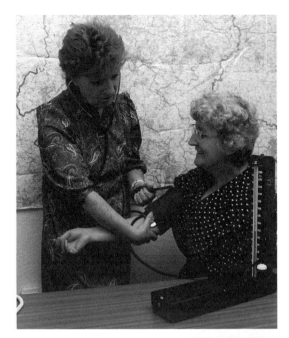

Checking blood pressure

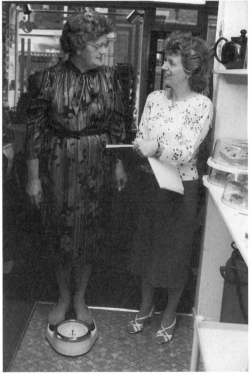

Monitoring weight

How did people hear about the shop?

A consideration of how people got to hear about the shop, and the frequency with which they visited, is a necessary prerequisite to discussing what people actually did, not least because what people did was related, broadly speaking, to whether or not they were first-time visitors or more regular customers. In terms of the criterion of accessibility, data from the census weeks and from the short response forms highlight the importance both of word-of-mouth and of having a physical location which is easily accessible to people who were often in Hanley doing other things. Word-of-mouth has come to play an increasingly important role as the project has developed. By the final year of the initial funding period, one-half of customers came through this means, while about one-third of customers find their way into the shop simply because they are 'just passing by'. Information on the local radio has consistently brought in about one in ten customers, while knowledge via the local press has become rather less influential over time.

With respect to the frequency of visits, it is no surprise to find that the proportion of first-time visitors has declined over the years. From a high of over 50 per cent at the first census in March 1987, the proportion settled down towards the end of that year at about one in five. This was then maintained over the greater part of the initial funding period. In effect, this meant that in an 'average' week when the shop was welcoming between 200 and 250 people, between 40 and 50 would have been visiting for the first time. This proportion of 'first-timers' began to show a slight drop at the last census, and in recent years has levelled out at around 10 per cent.

Information and choice at the Senior Health Shop

Very few people came to the shop merely just to have a look; having refreshments on offer was clearly a strong attraction. Over half of our respondents came to sample the 'healthy eating snacks' in the first full year of operation, with over one-third more combining refreshment with other activity. It was also our hope that even if people came solely to have a drink or snack of some kind, the fact that they were surrounded by health information would catch their interest. There is an indication from our data that, over time, more people did indeed combine refreshment taking with other things. These 'other things' have included picking up leaflets to take away, talking with workers or volunteers in the shop, having their weight monitored or blood pressure checked, and engaging in private advice sessions.

In particular, there has been a marked growth in verbal interaction between customers and staff. On average, just over half the customers during the first year sought advice from staff, but this rose dramatically to four out of five respondents during the last year of the initial funding. Accessing information by means of leaflet-taking also shows a similar pattern of growth, with about half the respondents taking leaflets in the first year, and three-quarters in subsequent years. Both these methods of acquiring information (in verbal and written form) were considered to be particularly important as a way of equipping older people with the means to make informed choices about their health. It is important to note here though that from March 1988 our questionnaires were modified to a self-completion format, and it is possible that customers may have overestimated the extent of both their verbal contact with staff, and their taking of leaflets. Nonetheless, these increases also reflect the conscious efforts in these directions being made by staff at the time, in order to try and counteract people using the shop simply as a café.

In addition to the data from the questionnaires, weekly reports from the Senior Health Shop also record the numbers of customers requesting personal advice sessions, and having weight and blood pressure checks – services on offer from staff and volunteers. Weight monitoring was (and indeed still is) the most popular service, with almost one in ten customers availing themselves of this opportunity. The late spring and early summer months (April to July) proved to be peak times, perhaps indicating that the desire to 'get into shape' and 'lose a few pounds' for the summer is still an important concern for some of the older people with whom we were in contact. However, it was never the project's intention to provide diet sheets to shop customers. Rather, staff would monitor a person's weight and discuss with the customer what she or he might need to do in terms of following a balanced diet, and/or combining this with suitable activity or exercise.

On average, 4 per cent of customers sought confidential health advice from a member of staff or one of the peer health counsellors. Although the shop is extremely small it is possible to conduct these consultations either in the CareLine office, or in an adjacent partitioned-off area. This affords greater privacy to customers than is possible through just talking with them while they are taking refreshments. A small percentage of customers (3 per cent) also had their blood pressure checked, with slight post-Christmas and post-Easter peaks discernible in these data. Again though, this was essentially a monitoring service provided by the shop manager who was herself a trained nurse. Customers would be given a slip of paper with the date, time and blood pressure reading, and would be encouraged to seek further advice from their general practitioner if the reading indicated that this might be necessary.

In this manner, it was possible for people to participate in activities which provided some way for them to check out various aspects of their own health, without the necessity of having to make a special appointment. They could also combine this with a visit to Hanley perhaps for other shopping on a regular basis.

Health information

Customers were interested in a whole variety of health issues. Again, the census data and the short response forms give us clear indications about what most interested these older people. Diet, exercise and weight are of concern to sizeable proportions of customers, followed by interests in stress control and in specific conditions. Over the initial funding period, only about one in six people (16 per cent) claimed that there was nothing in particular that interested them about health.

At the beginning of the project, two-fifths of respondents were interested in issues around diet and eating healthy foods. This proportion rose steadily over the next two years such that over half of respondents were expressing an interest in this area by the end of the initial funding period (this level of interest has been maintained in subsequent years). Concern with weight has shown a similar pattern of increasing interest, while exercise has been a consistent concern of approximately one in six respondents, and stress control and relaxation of one in eight people. Perhaps it is not altogether surprising that diet and weight feature so clearly in an environment where a 'healthy eating cafeteria' has been established as the primary means of attracting customers. However, what is also worthy of note is the growth in numbers of people who are 'generally interested' in health issues (from 10 per cent at the start to about 33 per cent currently) and the concomitant decline in concern over a specific condition. This point will be considered further below, when we examine the role of the shop in relation to more formal health services.

The Senior Health Shop: its impact on older people

Given these professed interests in health issues, the next logical step in the action research process was to try to determine whether contact with the shop had any effect whatsoever on health-related behaviours. The questionnaires asked people whether visiting the shop had made them think more about their health, or take some positive action (or indeed both). A further open-ended question invited them to describe in their own words what particular changes, if any, they had made or might be thinking about making.

Not surprisingly, first-time visitors to the shop responded to these questions largely in terms of what they intended to do, or would like to do. Obviously, not all of these people were actively thinking in this way but, as a general rule, between one-quarter and one-third of them were prepared to indicate possible changes they might make. By way of contrast, those who had visited over a period of time, perhaps talked with staff and volunteers as indicated above, and picked up and read a variety of literature, were able to tell us what concrete changes they had made. Between a half and two-thirds of this group indicated ways in which they had been able to take some positive action regarding their health.

In order to illustrate these intentions and actions Figure 7.1 provides details of comments made by respondents. It is evident from these remarks that people have begun to use the available information and support on offer in order to be able to make some real choices about various options which may be open to them concerning their health. The criterion of informed choice involves having a knowledge of the alternatives, as well as the means to put these choices into effect. Clearly, a proportion of our respondents are indeed exercising these choices.

What is also evident from our qualitative data are the ways in which change in one area sometimes begets further change. Having once successfully exercised such a choice, it perhaps becomes easier to do more. Consider Doris Battersby for example. Doris was 75 years of age and single. She had retired from a grocery shop, and was living alone in a semi-detached house in an area about one mile away, and surviving on a basic state pension (less than £50 per week). She first came alone to the shop soon after it opened, having seen it

HEALTH INTENTIONS	HEALTHY ACTIONS
Diet/healthy food/weight:	
'I'm thinking about making changes to my diet'	'I now eat less meat, more fish, and use wholemeal flour'
'I have high cholesterol and want to change my diet'	'I've cut down on fat, cakes and chocolate, and am eating more fruit, vegetables and wholemeal bread'
'I need to think more about what I eat'	'I eat less sugar and have decaffeinated coffee'
'I want to eat more fibre'	'I had wholemeal scones here and liked them, so I now buy wholemeal flour not white flour'
	'I've joined the weekly weigh-in'
Exercise/activity:	
'I'm thinking about trying a new activity'	'I've joined the Look After Yourself class at the Senior Centre'
'I want to do more exercise, but I don't know exactly what yet'	'I now exercise at home each morning and walk half an hour each day'
	'I've started dancing'
'I'd like to take up swimming'	'I'm taking swimming lessons and am into my third month'
'I want to go walking or rambling'	'I've joined the Beth Johnson ramblers, do yoga and keep fit'
Stress control/relaxation:	
'I'm thinking about ways to deal with my stress'	'I took up yoga after coming here, and find the relaxation is good for my Parkinson's disease'
'I want to learn how to overcome stress problems'	'I'm joining a relaxation class later this month'
	'I've joined the ramblers' club, and the walks have helped me in handling stress'

Figure 7.1   Healthy intentions and healthy actions

written about in the local press. She was 'generally interested' in health, but rated her own health as 'poor'. She subsequently became a 'regular', usually visiting about once a fortnight to 'take refreshment and browse among the literature'. A questionnaire interview with her during one census week recorded that, as a result of visiting the shop, she had made changes in a number of areas. She wrote: 'I now read more about health. I eat more wholemeal bread and have reduced sugar, salt and fat. I do keep fit at home, and I try to relax'.

Or perhaps Maureen Shaw: having recently retired from her job as a school secretary, Maureen heard about the shop from a friend. Then aged 62, she was married and living about one and a half miles away. Her income was under £100 per week. She too was 'generally interested' in health, and in swimming and walking. Her own health was 'good', and she called into the shop whenever she was in Hanley. She came alone, to 'take refreshment and browse', talk with the staff and pick up leaflets. She described the changes she had made to her diet and activity, and what she would still like to do:

> I eat less fat, practically no sugar and less fried food. I now walk about ten miles a week with the Ramblers' Association, swim once or twice a week, and paint with the local Water Colour Society. I would like to do something about my stress levels but find classes a bit expensive at the moment, as I have other activities.

Len White, a 69-year-old retired biscuit placer (in a pottery factory), had been coming to the shop since it opened in the summer of 1986. He was 'just passing by' but knew about, and was interested in, the work of the Beth Johnson Foundation. Living with his wife about half a mile away, on a basic state pension, they both visited once a month or less. He was interested in diet and in exercise, as well as in finding out more about diabetes, and rated his health as 'good'. He has picked up leaflets and spoken with the staff, and has thought about various aspects of his health since coming to the shop. When interviewed he explained how

> I have changed over to a high fibre diet. I exercise every morning and have bought a bouncer [a small trampoline]. I do pottery, and until Beth Johnson started swimming recently in Tunstall, there was none available at the northern end of the city.

Our final example in this section is Doreen Wilson. A 52-year-old housewife, she lived with her husband and son in a terraced house not half a mile from the city centre. Their household's total weekly income is less than £150 per week. Doreen was 'just passing by' and because she suffered with arthritis she came in 'to see if any leaflets could help me, and to ask advice about it regarding diet, exercise etc'. She usually came in on her own when she was in town and, in addition to arthritis, was 'generally interested' in health. She rated her own health as 'fair'. At the time we interviewed her, she had been visiting the shop for about two years. She wrote:

> Since being in the shop, I have completely changed from white bread to wholemeal. I do not take as much sugar, and do not use as much fat. I take care to watch my diet far more than previously. I go to swimming weekly, and have joined a social club once weekly which I enjoy. I am also now involved in running an elderly people's club in the area I live.

While one might want to argue that people may well have made these changes to their lifestyles without the shop, its presence and accessibility have provided a much needed and appreciated spur to some customers.

We come finally in this discussion about the shop to a consideration of what older people felt about it as a facility. Here, we were interested in what people liked about the shop, and how it compared with other more conventional health services such as clinics or visiting the doctor. To begin with, respondents at each census were asked to indicate what they liked best about the shop. The friendliness of the staff and the availability of good food have proved to be key. By the end of the initial funding period, in excess of 90 per cent of customers were commenting on the friendliness of staff, while two-thirds of respondents liked the good food. In recent years too, both these features are still singled out by the overwhelming majority of customers, as the reputation of the shop has continued to grow. Meanwhile, the attractive appearance of the shop has been one of its most enduring features, while the availability of information has come to be increasingly appreciated (only 10 per cent of respondents noted this as important in the early years, compared with about half currently).

The things which people like about the shop also seem to be very closely related to the things they say when asked to compare it with more formal health services. This open-ended question yielded a wide variety of responses which are collated together (by sex) in Table 7.2. Friendliness, food and information appear again here, together with important observations about the greater time which people have to discuss health matters; the fact that it is possible to 'call in' without an appointment (an aspect particularly valued by the men); and the unthreatening atmosphere. Given that the shop custom is dominated by women, it is particularly interesting to note that they (much more so than the men) feel that it is easier to sit and talk in the shop, both because staff have the time and because there are women present. In order to illustrate the variety of these responses, a selection of the comments made by respondents as they relate to the categories in Table 7.2 are given in Figure 7.2.

Conclusion

The Self Health Care in Old Age Project was never established with the aim of being a substitute for formal health services. Nor does it provide an 'alternative medicine source'. Rather, the data indicate that older people make use of the shop for a number of very positive reasons: they find it attractive and welcoming; they like the fact that it is specifically aimed at people over the age of 50; and the staff have the time and inclination to discuss health issues which older people themselves deem to be important. The ease of access it provides, and the information which is available have, we would contend, meant that the awareness, knowledge, understanding and competence of many of our customers has been raised. In fact, when asked, only 10 per cent of respondents say they can think of anywhere else to go to obtain similar

Table 7.2 Comparison of the Senior Health Shop with more formal health services

	Women		Men		Total
	n	*(%)*	*n*	*(%)*	*n*
Friendly; relaxed; informal	207	(32)	60	(36)	267
Time to talk; easy to talk; women present	201	(31)	20	(12)	221
Easy to obtain leaflets; information	136	(21)	28	(17)	164
No appointment needed	91	(14)	42	(25)	133
Unthreatening	97	(15)	20	(12)	117
Food available	45	(7)	20	(12)	65
Other	26	(4)	5	(3)	31
Base (n)	648		166		814

Friendly; relaxed; informal:
'It's much more friendly and it seems to me, on my first visit, that the staff are very helpful'
'The approach is very caring, enabling me to open out more'
'It's a friendly atmosphere and you can get advice without feeling a nuisance'
'It's more free and easy, and informal'

Time to talk; easy to talk; women present:
'The staff are willing to sit and talk – not like the GP's, where you're in and out with a written prescription'
'You have more time to be able to talk. Doctors write prescriptions before they know what you've got, and you feel as if you're taking up someone else's time'
'It's more free and easy, and you're more likely to tell people how you feel, and be able to discuss things more fully'
'It's less formal and easier to discuss problems'
'More women can talk in a shop like this'
'It's women here, and you can't talk to doctors because most of them are men'

Easy to obtain leaflets; information:
'There's readily available information, in a pleasant and quiet atmosphere'
'Information and leaflets are available and you're not pestered by anyone'
'You're able just to take leaflets'

No appointment needed:
'GPs are very busy, but you can call in anytime here'
'You have to make a definite effort and appointment to go to a doctor's, but here you can pop in when you've done some shopping and have a nice chat with the staff if you're worried about anything'
'There are no waiting lists here and you can come in when you want'

Unthreatening:
'The relaxed manner of staff means people are not afraid to talk to them'
'I'm not frightened to come in here and talk, but I am frightened to go to the doctor's'
'I wouldn't be frightened to ask questions here'

Figure 7.2   Comments about the Senior Health Shop

kinds of health information and advice. For the majority, this would be their GP. There are implications from our findings for the ways in which health promoting information and activities are offered to older people – an issue to which we shall return in the concluding chapter. In the mean time, these final two comments from customers illustrate most graphically the complementary nature of the shop:

It's a good start because you can walk in, look round and walk out again if you want to, but it does start you thinking.

It feels like a half-way house before going to the GP – for self-help rather than drugs.

8

Self health care in action: skills development and empowerment among older people

Introduction

This chapter moves on to a consideration of how, once older people have gained access and begun to participate in activities such as those provided under the auspices of the Self Health Care in Old Age Project, they begin to develop and build upon particular interests and skills. This discussion is illustrated by reference to the variety of health-related activities designed to facilitate and encourage self health care practices among older people. More particularly, we draw on information from the records we maintained relating to the Look After Yourself courses held at the Senior Centre, and to the research we conducted with these participants.

The LAY courses were begun as a direct response to the growth of interest in health-related matters noted in Chapter 5. Fortunately, the Foundation already had facilities for people to pursue activities in the form of both the Leisure Association and the Senior Centre. Since it was our belief that there was little point in encouraging and advising people to adopt healthier life-styles if no information was available on how to achieve this, or no facilities were offered to do so, it was logical that where possible, we should be able to respond constructively to practical suggestions about additional courses or activities.

The discussion below is based on feedback culled from course monitoring forms; from 'open response paragraphs' written by course participants; from participant and non-participant observation of the courses; and from focus group interviews held with participants (see Table 6.1). It should also be noted here that slight alterations were made to course feedback forms over the period of time the project was funded. However, the basic core information obtained remained the same and included socio-demographic data; how people heard about the course; what their motivations for joining were; changes in health behaviour/status as a result of participation on the course; future intentions; and an indication of what participants felt they had gained.

Participation in the LAY courses

The first ten-week LAY course was held between April and June 1986 (prior to the opening of the Senior Health Shop). It was tutored by a lecturer seconded from a local further education (FE) college and, following the success of the first course, it became a regular feature of the Senior Centre programme on Friday mornings. Participants engaged in a three-part programme based on the then Health Education Council's new national scheme. The programme had been modified by the FE lecturer for use with people over the age of 50, and included first, a period of exercise; second, a period of relaxation; and third, discussion of particular health issues. In total, a session would last approximately one and a half hours. Participants were taught how to monitor their own pulse and to exercise within a range suited to their own individual capabilities. They also learnt a variety of relaxation techniques.

Who got involved?

The initial course was an all female affair, with fourteen women aged from 57 to 68 taking part. Three of these original fourteen women decided to continue with the course when a new one began the following October. Nineteen people enrolled for the second course, although three were unable to commence it due to other commitments. This pattern, of some people dropping out and other new people joining, was repeated over the first two years that the course ran. Each course usually had between fifteen and twenty participants and, after the first course, there have always been one or two men as well.

In addition, not everyone completed feedback forms. This was a voluntary activity, and some people either did not have the time or perhaps did not attend the last session when these were usually given out. Consequently, during the first two years of the courses, we have information from a total of thirty participants. Some of these individuals have attended regularly for a number of years, and this aspect is discussed further below. However, it is important to observe here that it was never the intention to have LAY courses which people continued to attend. Where they had been run elsewhere, and with other age groups, they were designed as a one-off basic introduction to health issues. Our experience was that once people had got a taste for exercise, relaxation and discussion, a growing number wanted to continue with it on a regular basis and within some kind of external framework such as the course provided. As a result, graduates of the basic course, which ran for the first two years, lobbied to have an additional course. This was eventually fitted in before yoga on a Friday morning (see Chapter 5) and, subsequently, two courses have run now for many years.

Looking at the data which we have on these thirty participants reveals that

Table 8.1 LAY participants by age

	Female		Male		Totals	
	n	*(%)*	*n*	*(%)*	*n*	*(%)*
Age 50–9	4	(18)	–	–	4	(15)
Age 60–9	17	(77)	4	(80)	21	(78)
Age 70 plus	1	(5)	1	(20)	2	(7)
Totals	22	(100)	5	(100)	27	(100)

women outnumbered men by five to one: there were twenty-five women (83 per cent) and five men (17 per cent). These proportions are very similar to the shop data (see Table 7.2) and reveal the continuing attraction of such health related opportunities for older women.

In terms of the age distribution of participants, Table 8.1 shows that nearly four-fifths of people were in their sixties. Apart from one man who was aged 72, the other four were in their mid-sixties (aged 64–7). The women, by contrast, covered a 20-year age span: the youngest participant was 54 and the oldest 74. Although three women declined to give their age, the LAY courses seem, on the whole, to have attracted a narrower age cohort than the shop.

Turning to consider the marital status of participants, we see from Table 8.2 that over half of the women were widowed compared with only one man in this situation. Conversely, the men were married and tended, interestingly, to come as a couple with their wives. This may say something about the image of health-related courses and is a point to which we shall return in the concluding chapter. While the data on men's marital status compare closely with the men who used the shop, a higher proportion of the women who came to the LAY courses are widows (52 per cent compared with 43 per cent). Again, this may indicate that these women were looking for things in addition to partaking in a health course.

Twenty-five participants provided information about their employment status prior to retirement (five women declined to answer this question). In keeping with the area's tradition of female employment, fourteen (70 per cent) had worked, one regarded herself as unemployed and five (25 per cent) had been housewives. All five men had worked, three in skilled manual occupations and two in professions. The women, by contrast, had been employed

Table 8.2 LAY participants by marital status

	Female		Male		Totals	
	n	*(%)*	*n*	*(%)*	*n*	*(%)*
Married	10	(44)	4	(80)	14	(50)
Widowed	12	(52)	1	(20)	13	(46)
Single	1	(4)	–	–	1	(4)
Totals	23	(100)	5	(100)	28	(100)

across a range of occupational categories, varying from unskilled jobs such as shop assistants, cleaners and doing café work, to skilled clerical and technical jobs, and professional occupations such as nursing. The LAY courses, like the shop, were not solely the preserve of middle-class older people but tended to attract a spectrum of participants.

How then did people get to hear about the courses? One participant had seen the course advertised at another class she attended, twelve had heard about it by word-of-mouth (41 per cent), nine via the Senior Centre itself (31 per cent) and four while visiting the shop (14 per cent).

Skills development on the LAY courses

The most obvious practical skill which people learnt through their participation was how to take their own pulse rate, before and after exercising. Everyone was taught how to do this. Some participants began the course with a very low level of fitness and stamina; others had had – or indeed were to experience – various forms of surgery, including heart surgery, hip replacements and so on, which meant that they needed to exercise a degree of caution over what and how much they did. Others were on different kinds of medication, including some to help control blood pressure, which meant that pulse rates would be lower. Consequently, with the help of the tutor, it was possible for each individual to exercise at a safe level, one which would enable him or her to achieve maximum benefit. Being able to estimate one's health status in this way is one of the basic diagnostic self health care skills noted by Coppard and his colleagues (1984) and discussed earlier in Chapter 3.

Participants also became knowledgeable about how their own health status and different kinds of exercise would affect their pulse rate. For example, Mavis Fuller (aged 62) wrote: 'One week I wasn't too well because I had a cold. This meant my pulse rate went up that week. At other times though, I could do more time on the exercises each week before my pulse went up.'

Emily Davidson (aged 61) was aware that 'The wall press-ups and the bench steps were more strenuous and would put my pulse rate up', while Edna Lockett (aged 59) commented that: 'The more I do, the more time I can do on each exercise before my pulse changes'. This ability to be able to exercise for longer without becoming breathless was noticed by many of the participants, women and men alike.

Health promoting skills

Furthermore, the LAY courses directly addressed one key area in the development of older people's self health care skills, namely those skills relating to health promotion and disease prevention (Coppard *et al.* 1984). Exercise, diet and the development, encouragement and support needed to choose and then maintain a healthy lifestyle were all integral to these courses. Over and above these dimensions though, the course also placed emphasis on good mental health and the teaching of relaxation techniques to help alleviate stress and tension. In order to explore whether or not people had been helped to learn or enhance these kinds of skills, participants were asked whether or not they had noticed any change in their health or well-being since starting the course. If they responded affirmatively, they were then asked to explain what these changes had been and how they related to four areas: diet, physical health, stress management and general mood.

All five men responded affirmatively, as did nineteen (79 per cent) women. In Table 8.3, we can see in which areas people felt that the course had had most impact. Of the twenty-nine participants who responded, over two-thirds were aware of a change in their mood: all of the men, and fifteen of the women. This was followed by a majority of both men and women who noted improvements in managing stress and tension. Dietary changes and improvements to one's physical stamina or suppleness were experienced by nearly half the participants, and there are some indications of interesting variations between men and women in these responses.

In order to illustrate the variety of these responses, a selection of the comments made by respondents as they relate to the categories in Table 8.3 are given in Figure 8.1.

These comments illustrate both the varied dimensions to health noted and discussed in earlier chapters, as well as the benefits of combining opportunities for physical exercise with relaxation and discussion time. This is an example of an holistic approach to the health needs of older participants, an approach which addresses emotional as well as physical aspects of health, and which acknowledges the importance too of the social dimension. The LAY course has given participants structure and purpose in their lives, and something to look forward to, as well as enabling them to 'feel better'.

What did people do with what they had learnt?

Learning certain health-related skills is all very well, but leading a healthier lifestyle is as much about maintenance as it is about acquiring the skills initially. Consequently, participants in the courses were asked whether they intended to continue with the new patterns of behaviour once the course was over and, if so, what these patterns of behaviour would be related to. They were also asked whether they intended to join any other groups or classes as a result of attending the Look After Yourself course.

Table 8.3 Health changes since start of LAY course

	Female		Male		Totals	
	n	*(%)*	*n*	*(%)*	*n*	*(%)*
Improved mood	15	(63)	5	(100)	20	(69)
Management of stress/tension	14	(58)	4	(80)	18	(62)
Dietary changes	10	(42)	4	(80)	14	(48)
Physical stamina or suppleness	11	(46)	2	(40)	13	(45)
Other changes	5	(21)	1	(20)	6	(21)
Base n	24	(100)	5	(100)	29	(100)

Improved mood:
'I'm calmer I think'   'I'm more relaxed'
'I'm more hopeful'   'I'm happy'
'I'm more well balanced'   'I feel much better'
'I think I cope better'   'My mood has improved generally'
'I'm more even tempered'   'I have more confidence'

Management of stress/tension:
'I'm learning how to manage my stress   'I'm much better at managing my
  and tension'   stress'
'I get rid of tension easier and I relax 'I am able to relax much more easily
  better'   now'

Dietary changes:
'My diet is better'   'I eat less fattening foods'
'I eat more sensibly now'   'I've lost eight pounds in weight'
'I eat less fats'

Physical stamina or suppleness:
'I'm much more supple now as it has   'I don't get tired as quickly as I used
  taught me the right way to exercise'   to'
'I can do more now, and walk a lot   'I feel much better and am able to walk
  further than when I first came'   better'
'It's less of an effort to exercise now' 'I now feel fit'

Other changes:
'I like the company'   'It's nice to be able to chat to people'
'I now sleep well'   'It's something to look forward to'

Figure 8.1   Comments on health changes since start of LAY course

All twenty-nine participants who responded to these questions did so affirmatively, and the areas they intended to go on addressing are shown in Table 8.4.

A substantial majority of participants indicated that they intended to continue with what they had learnt in relation to exercise, the management of

Table 8.4   Health intentions following participation in LAY course

	Female		Male		Totals	
	n	*(%)*	*n*	*(%)*	*n*	*(%)*
Exercise	17	(71)	2	(40)	19	(66)
Management of stress/tension	14	(58)	3	(60)	17	(59)
Dietary changes	13	(54)	3	(60)	16	(55)
Join a new group or activity	9	(38)	2	(40)	11	(38)
Continue with LAY group	7	(29)	1	(20)	8	(28)
Base n	24	(100)	5	(100)	29	(100)

Exercise:

'I'll carry on exercising'
'I'll do daily, longer walks'
'I'll do ten minutes each day'

'I'll do more exercise at home'
'I'll try to remember some gentle exercises each day'

Management of stress/tension:

'I shall try harder with this'
'I shall try to be calmer'

'I will practise relaxation at home'
'I will try to relax daily'

Dietary changes:

'I will continue to eat better and try and lose weight'
'I'm not going to eat chocolate bars'
'I aim to lose a stone in weight'

'I have changed my way of eating and will stick with this'
'I shall try and eat less'
'We'll carry on with the new pattern of eating less fats and more fibre'

Join a new group or activity:

'Join a keep-fit class'
'Take up swimming again/learn to swim'
'Rambling with the Beth Johnson Foundation'
'Start painting again/ join an art class'

'Join a relaxation class'
'Dancing/learning to dance'
'I would like to try Tai Chi Chuan'

Figure 8.2 Comments on health intentions following LAY course

stress and tension, and dietary changes. The women in particular were keen to continue with physical activity. About one in three people were prompted to consider joining another kind of group or class, and about one in four wanted to continue doing a further LAY course. Examples of the kinds of things that participants intended to continue doing are shown in Figure 8.2.

These comments again illustrate the range of things that people were now beginning to think about in relation to maintaining their health status. They had acquired certain additional self health care skills which, together with the increased knowledge and information they now had to hand, enabled them to make some choices about their future activity. For some, there were very clearly defined goals such as wanting to lose weight; for others, the course was the spur for them to perhaps take up something again which they had not done for a while; for others still, there had opened up the possibility of learning and experiencing something completely new.

Indeed, following on from the success of the LAY courses, we noted in Chapter 6 that other related courses were subsequently put on at the Senior Centre in order to respond to the expressed wishes of many older people for further opportunities to engage in health-related activities. The LAY tutor agreed to offer two courses: one on diet and nutrition, and one on stress management. These three courses supplemented the already extensive programme of activities offered under the auspices of the Senior Centre and the Leisure Association (see Chapter 5).

What is also worthy of note here in respect of skills' development is that the graduates of the first LAY courses were faced in the summer of 1987 with the prospect of their tutor not being available to lead the course (her college commitments and contract did not allow for her to continue over the summer vacation period). In response, the group decided that they were sufficiently skilled and confident to continue leading the courses themselves. This has happened on a number of subsequent occasions when there have been possible hiatuses because of a change of tutor, or while tutors have been away on holiday or ill. This clearly demonstrates how some participants, once they have acquired sufficient skill and confidence, are enabled to become effective leaders for their peers. It also brings us, in the final section of this chapter, to a consideration of whether these kinds of changes lead to a sense of empowerment among the older people who come into contact with the project.

Self-empowered health behaviour: reality or illusion?

Although the older people encountered in the previous pages may well not apply the term 'empowered' to the changes they have made, many of them certainly demonstrate raised awareness, increased knowledge and understanding, and greater competence in health-related behaviours. These are clear signs of empowerment (see Chapter 3). This applies to people who came into the shop, many of whom gathered information, talked with staff and volunteers and, as a result, then went on to find out more, join other classes or groups, change their diets and so on. In addition, it will be remembered that some of the participants in Look After Yourself were involved in a number of courses. In fact, thirteen of our sample attended two or more courses over the first two years. Between them, they illustrate something of the incremental process by which health promotion is achieved and then maintained.

In order to help answer the question of whether self-empowered health behaviour is a reality or illusion, we consider five individual stories. All five took part in the LAY courses but this is not all they eventually did. We shall meet three widows – Mary Riley, Sarah Bagshot and June Marshall – as well as Bert Diamond, a married man, and Daisy Clifton, a married woman. The illustrations are based primarily on information from feedback forms, focus group interviews, paragraphs which participants wrote about the courses and from participant observation (see Table 6.1). In Daisy Clifton's case, she was also one of the small sample who were interviewed in depth about their lives and experiences of health and illness.

Mary Riley attended the first LAY course in the early summer of 1986. She had been a nurse and was now, at the age of 60, a widow. She read about the course in one of the local papers and decided to come along and find out what it involved. Although she had a general interest in health, she did not have anyone she felt she could talk to about her health worries and thought the course might help. The possibility of making new friends, and the fact that the course provided something for her own age group that was more than just bingo and a chat, were also attractive.

A small frail woman, who suffered with arthritis, Mary seemed to have great difficulty initially with the physical exercises. However, she greatly enjoyed all the sessions on that first course and noted on her feedback questionnaire that, in terms of her general mood, 'I am happy while I'm at the

Senior Centre'. Diet also concerned her and, as a result of participating in the first course, she wrote that 'I now eat potatoes with the skins on'.

Her awareness of diet, and what constitutes a healthy diet, continued to improve over the subsequent courses she attended. She wrote: 'I am more conscious of the importance of a low salt, low sugar and low fat diet, and of having a high fibre content' and she went on to note later that 'I am now aware of how to avoid sugars and fats, and I include bran in my diet'. Her mood and her ability to deal with stress and tension also evidenced change. By the end of the second course, she wrote: 'I now do deep breathing exercises and have begun to cry instead of suppressing it. I find it as important as laughter'.

A year after first joining the LAY courses, a group interview records this comment from one of Mary's co-participants: 'When we first started, you had a problem with your arm and your collar bone. Now you feel better and look better. Mentally, you seem to have a different outlook'. Mary herself was acutely aware of these changes. Another of her feedback forms records that the most important thing she gained from the course was that 'I am a happier person and am more outgoing', while a paragraph she subsequently wrote highlights the importance of a mutually supportive environment: 'I enjoy coming for the company and, best of all, the tutor makes everyone feel as if they are a real person. We all look forward to the next session, and the next course, and I have benefited both mentally and physically'.

Coming to the LAY course made Mary feel that she could do something positive about her health. Although her arthritis continued to trouble her, she found that she developed more stamina and recorded that 'I can do longer periods of exercise'. At home, she tried 'to remember to do some gentle exercise each day'. Early on, she signalled her intention to take up rambling, which she subsequently did. This was followed by wanting to learn to dance, and then to learn to swim. These too she achieved and, when last spoken with, her next project was to take up photography. In sum, Mary felt that the courses gave her a little more self-confidence and helped her feel better about herself.

Our second widow is *Sarah Bagshot*. Sarah was 57 when she joined the first course and had been a housewife and a school dinner lady. She heard about it from a friend and, like Mary, was generally interested in health but wanted to learn more about what she could do to keep herself healthy. She was a large, matronly woman who told us that 'the doctor ordered me to lose weight'. Although she had modified her diet and was eating 'health foods', she felt 'I was eating too much of it. For example, the leaflets said one and a half ounces of porridge, but I think I was having three ounces'. Sarah was also aware that exercise would help, but she found this hard to do on her own and thought a course might encourage her. Being widowed, she also felt that she did not really have anyone to whom she could talk about her health worries, so making new friends and contacts was also part of Sarah's motivation for coming to the course.

By the end of the first ten weeks, Sarah was able to record that her physical stamina and suppleness was a 'lot better' and that she was 'getting benefit from eating better and losing weight'. Through her attendance at subsequent

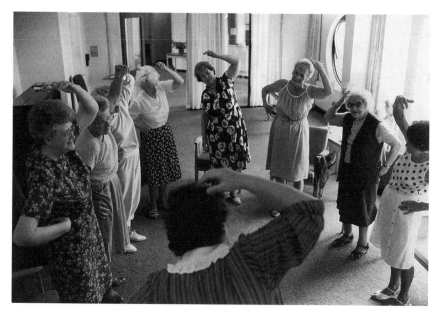

A gentle exercise and discussion group

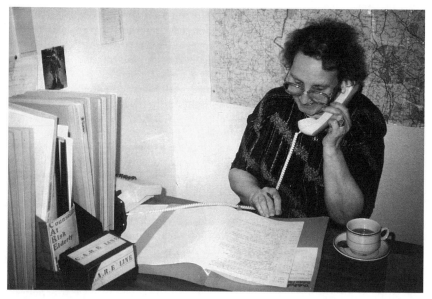

CareLine volunteer at work

courses she went on to find that 'I can manage to do more exercises'. Later still she was able to be more specific about these improvements, writing that 'I now have much more movement in my knees and can move my neck much better'. A paragraph she wrote after a year of attendance also records these changes, as well as indicating Sarah's awareness of the importance of the social interaction which is an integral part of the course: 'I really enjoy coming here. I am not a good mixer but I do enjoy being with you all. Also, my knees and feet bend a lot better with the exercises we do. I look forward to every Friday'.

Although Sarah concentrated over the earlier courses on exercise and diet, she was also aware that her ability to manage tension and stress was 'not good'. This frustrated her and she noted that 'I need to try harder with this part of the course'. After two years she felt that she was beginning to get somewhere with this element too. In response to a question about what she had found particularly interesting, she wrote: 'the relaxation, because I have just managed to do it after a long time! I'm getting better at it'. Indeed, this achievement, combined with a sense that the course made her feel that she could do something positive about her health, and that it had given her a lot more self-confidence, led her to express an interest in trying Tai Chi Chuan. Sarah continued with the courses, lost the weight she wanted to and wrote in testimony that 'I can only say it's saved my life'.

June Marshall, another widow, expressed similar sentiments. June was introduced to the course by having heard about it at the shop. The peer health counsellor who had talked with her brought her along to the start of the second course. A housewife aged 60, June had been recently widowed and came across the shop while in Hanley one day. She was generally interested in health, and was a fit looking woman for whom dancing had been a passion earlier in life. She had been devastated by the loss of her husband, was on tranquillizers prescribed for her by her doctor, but was also aware that she needed to find something which would give her a sense of purpose and meaning.

She recorded that 'I was in a bad state' but, by the end of her first ten weeks on the course, she had already begun to notice changes. About her mood and her management of stress and tension, she wrote: 'I think I cope better with this aspect of myself. I no longer feel the need of the Valium type pills pre-scribed for me'. Indeed, she felt that the most important things she had gained from the course were that 'I look and feel better in myself, both mentally and physically'.

June's mental state grew more positive with each successive course. She attended keep-fit classes, indicated a desire to take up swimming again, and was interested, like Sarah, in learning Tai Chi. She also went on to become involved in social aspects of the Senior Centre and with the Leisure Associ-ation. Extracts from a series of paragraphs that she wrote illustrate most graphically the progress she made:

When I started this course, I was in a sad state due to losing my husband . . . The company of these wonderful people, the understanding of our instructor, plus the classes have made a big difference to my life. I feel more able to cope with things, and am now completely off the pills prescribed by my doctor.

. . . my first term as you know, I was in a very bad mental state. This time I am much more calm. I love the talks and videos. The discussions are very stimulating and the exercises are good as a lead up to relaxation which I enjoy.

. . . the course has made me think even more about my eating habits. I have tried for some years to eat healthily. Nevertheless, I have found this very constructive . . . the stress part is very helpful for myself. Also, to hear about other people's stresses and to discuss ways and means to allay them.

I have once again found this course very helpful in helping me improve my way of life. Each time I have found that the exercises, talks, relaxation, plus the company of lovely people, sets me up for days.

I have learned to live again . . . I hate to think how I might have been had I not joined the courses.

We turn now to consider *Bert Diamond* who, while perhaps not exhibiting such dramatic changes as the three widows, nonetheless found that the course helped particularly with his mood and mental well-being. At the time Bert joined the second course, he was aged 72 and a retired bricklayer. A small wiry man, he suffered badly with arthritis. Like the women, he was motivated to attend because he wanted to find out what he might do to keep healthy, but found exercising hard to do on his own. Although married, he also wanted to make new friends and contacts and, interestingly, wanted to gain more confidence in himself.

Like June, Bert found out about the course from a peer health counsellor he met while attending a yoga class at the Senior Centre. It was then not too big a step to also come to the LAY course. He described his first ten weeks as 'wonderful', and wrote: 'The class is wonderful. The exercises help a lot and the company is very good . . . I wouldn't miss it for anything'. He felt that it had taught him to eat better and he commented that he was now 'more relaxed'. As a result of attending, Bert decided that he would join another LAY course nearer to where he lived. This he did, and it is recorded in feedback from later courses.

Not until the end of his attendance at the second course do we get some indication of why Bert perhaps felt so unself-confident when he first started participating. He began, on the feedback form, to comment on the importance of the company to him and in a longer paragraph he wrote:

When I started I was in a bad way. My doctor had given me Opren tablets and I was in a very bad way. One specialist said I had a month to live. Since I started the classes I am wonderful. My joints are still very bad, but in myself I am very good. Our teacher is very good, and the company is lovely.

With the prospect of only a month to live hanging over him Bert had, understandably, held off from fully engaging with everyone in the early days. As he continued to improve, his confidence grew visibly. He had, he said, gained 'everything' from coming to the courses: they had made him feel he could do something positive about his health; improved his stamina a lot; made him a lot more aware about what he ate; helped him to relax more easily and, above all, given him a lot more self-confidence. He had plans to join a keep-fit class and to take up swimming, and resolved to practise and do more relaxation and exercise at home. He summed it all up by writing that: 'Friends tell me I look ten years younger, and I feel it'.

Our final story concerns *Daisy Clifton*. Daisy was interviewed at some length about her life and, in addition to information from feedback forms, group interviews and her own written comments, we have four hours of taped interview. She was 59 years of age when she joined the first LAY course, and 61 when she was personally interviewed. The seventh of eleven children, spanning 20 years between them, Daisy describes her early life as follows:

> I was brought up in a little terraced house with two bedrooms . . . we slept three in a bed. The rooms were quite big. You don't really think so in those terraced houses, but we used to have two double beds in both rooms, and a wardrobe . . . The toilet was down the garden . . . not too far from the back kitchen. We had coal fired heating, just downstairs . . . there were fire grates upstairs but we didn't have them. We didn't bother with them unless someone was ill, then we needed them.

With so many children to look after, her mother did not go to work. Her father worked in a factory which manufactured sanitary ware but, when Daisy was just 4 years old, he had an accident. She remembers that for many years he was unemployed until, in the mid-1930s, he went into the army 'to earn a bit of money'. When war broke out, he was too old to stay in, so he went to work in a munitions factory. He stayed on there after the Second World War until it closed down. He then worked at a place which sold building materials until he retired at the age of 75. Daisy recalls:

> Those were difficult times when dad was out of work – he must have been out of work for ten years . . . it was very hard. It must have been very difficult for mother to feed us all.

Nevertheless, she said, 'we were always happy'. Life for Daisy was framed by family, school and the church (they were Methodists). It was also punctuated by illness, both her own and that of other family members:

> Mother had a lot of sickness with all of us. I was seriously ill when I was 4. I had pneumonia. I went into hospital and I was unconscious for two weeks. They put me in a glass case. I can remember, before going into hospital . . . I was sitting on the pavement . . . and I remember looking down the street and I saw my friend Margaret crying at the bottom of the street because I was going into hospital . . . my brother had diphtheria. If one of us caught something, the rest would catch it as well.

When war broke out, she was 12. She missed quite a lot of schooling at about this time because 'all we did was knitting . . . knitting balaclavas for the forces'. Leaving school two years later at the age of 14, she now regrets that she had no qualifications at all and feels that 'I have missed out on a lot'. Wartime was also responsible, she feels, for the illnesses which plagued her adult life. They used to sleep every night in an air raid shelter:

> The condensation in there – I sometimes wonder if that's where we got the rheumatics from – was terrible . . . there was only a paraffin heater in there . . . The blankets were always sopping wet with condensation and they had to be dried every day on the line. You were lucky to get them dry. They used to get covered in soot from the factories . . . I think it was the air raid shelter that affected my health, and that's why I have arthritis. I'm sure that's why a lot of people suffer from it.

After she left school, Daisy went to work in a factory:

> a clay 'un . . . I did that till I was 20, then I went in the Naafi for 12 months. I served meals to the forces . . . then I went back home and worked in the factory.

> I met Reg on the factory, he was a saggar. I'd known him since I was 14. We went out when I was 17, then he went in the army. Then we got married when I was 22.

She goes on to describe her and Reg's working and family life which, while poor like her parents, was not overshadowed by unemployment or having a large family:

> I got married at 22, stayed and looked after my daughter till she was 5 years old, then went back to working in cafés. That's most of my life: cafés and canteens . . . Then I became a home help for eleven years.
>
> Reg has been mostly on the railway . . . he was a trackman. He's never been unemployed. As he left one job, he'd get another one. He's never been on strike, never had any broken periods. When you think of it – Dad unemployed all those years and how he coped. I just had one daughter . . . I felt as though I couldn't afford more children. I didn't really deep down want any more, financially. I used to be in fear of having any more.

She and Reg, apart from when they lived 'in rooms' when they were first married, have always lived in the council house they still rent on a large estate. As indicated above, Daisy's adult life has been punctuated by ill health:

> I have always had aches and pains and I had arthritis before I came into this house [25 years previously] . . . Healthwise, I have gone to work and been really ill. I've walked, even knowing that it was crippling me . . . I was first X-rayed over 20 years ago and they said I had arthritis in both hips and the base of the spine . . . Arthritis – I can never remember not having it.

The advice she received from her doctors was that 'I was too young to do anything about it'. She was told that hip replacement operations at the time would last for only about five years, 'so you tried to keep going as long as possible'. Keeping going meant that, over the years, Daisy was tried on a variety of different medications with various side-effects:

I've had my hands blow up with tablets, my legs swell up . . . I've been on strong pain killers. I've taken one before going to the chemist to fetch a prescription and I've had to come home before I finished my shopping. I was nearly knocked out for 24 hours with one kind . . . I can't remember the tablets I have had because I had so many of them.

Eventually, two years before the project and the LAY courses began, Daisy had her hip operation:

I was only in nine days. They reckoned I should have been in two weeks with having them both done. I was told I was the model patient. Two days after having them done my friends came to see me. I was just walking to the toilet on a walking frame and they said, 'Daisy, the pain's gone out of your face. All the pain you've had in your face for years has just literally gone'. To be free of pain is marvellous.

Daisy was keen to return to work so when she went for a check up: 'I asked the hospital what exercises I could do'. The response was disappointing to say the least: 'he said, "There's nothing we can give you. You know how far your limitations go, so no way can we tell you what to do". I felt a bit lost really because I didn't know what to do'.

She tried to return to her work as a home help, but found it impossible. The years of medication were also exerting their toll on her health. Twelve months after having her hips done, she had hepatitis followed closely by another operation, this time to remove her gall bladder. She then had problems with her pancreas:

Then they said it was my pancreas and that I was very lucky to be alive. I lost two stone in 15 weeks . . . they said it was the tube and it was very inflamed . . . I was in hospital 10 days the first time; the second time I was in 14 days, and the third time I was rushed in, I was in for three weeks . . . They must have unblocked the tube. I never asked them because I just felt too ill to ask. It took me another 12 months to pull myself together after that.

For Daisy, 'pulling herself together' led her to the Beth Johnson Foundation and the LAY course:

I first heard about it from the radio . . . they just told you to call the office for information. I decided to go and have a look . . . what attracted me was that it [the Senior Centre] was a club for the over 50s. When I went down and walked in, Dora [one of the peer health counsellors: see Chapter 9] said 'hello', and came and sat with me. She got talking to me, she was counselling me which I didn't know at the time . . . The Look After Yourself course had been going for two weeks before I joined it.

She joined in for the remaining weeks of that first course, and has been a regular and committed participant ever since. Her feedback forms recorded positive changes to her physical capabilities, to her stamina and to her mood. Two years after she began, she observed:

To me it was a new way of life. I couldn't do much exercise and going to that class, and doing simple exercises, I find it marvellous . . . I feel quite chuffed that I can raise my leg a bit further every time, because when I first went I couldn't lift it at all. That class, and my diet, has helped a lot. I even used to have arthritis in my neck as well, and doing them simple exercises has helped, and I feel it's doing me good.

Participation has also given her a lot more self-confidence: confidence to join in other activities and to make new friends. Daisy goes every Friday to the Senior Centre:

We have a period of discussion at the Look After Yourself course. I feel I have learned a lot off the people there . . . I think it has helped my confidence a lot. I go about 10.30 and join the class at 11. Our class goes on till 12.30. Then we have a meal and a good natter. I stay for the dance in the afternoon . . . I leave the Centre at 3.45 . . . The friends I have made I do meet outside.

. . . we go on day trips. There's about four or five of us and they'll say, 'Will we go for a meal?', and I'll say, 'How about a nice pub?' We have a look, and I always go in first and survey the place. I don't think I would have looked in a pub like that before . . . years ago I wouldn't even think of it . . . I can see the other women are a bit timid, so I put a brave face on.

Daisy always has, and still does, travel everywhere by bus because 'If I depended on Reg, I wouldn't go anywhere'. This independence is vitally important to her and as she says: 'I love sitting on the bus and looking at the countryside . . . to me, retirement is lovely so long as I can afford to go on these little things'. Her lifelong love of sewing now finds expression in work that she proudly exhibits at craft fairs and exhibitions, and she continues to knit (though not balaclavas!) and to tend her garden: 'I have plenty of things to occupy my mind'.

This self-confidence is also evident in her dealings with others, particularly health professionals. She says:

I ask more questions than I have ever done in my life. Before, I just took it that they knew what they were doing. I don't know why I never asked questions. I think I was shy. I used to think people might think I was being cocky or nosey if I asked questions . . . we are afraid to ask. Doctors are supposed to be superior in their field. I say to myself, they are only human beings, why should you be afraid of them?

Never, throughout the hours of in-depth interviews with Daisy, did she ever use the word 'empowered'. Yet her story graphically illustrates all that she has learnt and how her involvement with the courses and the project has enabled her to use these abilities. The final words of this chapter are, fittingly, hers:

The best thing that ever happened to me is the Beth Johnson. I have a different outlook on life, and I have met some beautiful friends. They aren't just casual friends, they are true friends . . . I haven't been on holiday for six years, and it won't bother me if I don't go on holiday again so long as I am healthy. I used to go on holiday, and Reg would have to wrap me up in blankets because of my arthritis, even if the sun was shining. I used to be glad to be home. Now I look at every day as being a holiday.

9

Self health care in action: its impact on volunteers and staff

Introduction

Having examined the project's impact in terms of the older people who became involved through the shop and the various health-related activities, we turn finally to consider what volunteers and staff both contributed and gained through their inclusion in the Self Health Care in Old Age Project. As in previous chapters, the present discussion examines these issues according to the criteria generated by the project itself – namely, participation, access, informed choice, skills development, and empowerment. Again, discussion here has, of necessity, to be selective. While Chapter 7 contained a lot of detailed information on the Senior Health Shop and Chapter 8 on the health-related courses and activities (notably the Look After Yourself course), the major focus here is on the peer health counselling and CareLine parts of the project (though where appropriate, volunteer work in the shop, the Senior Centre and on health-related activities will also be referred to).

In particular, we draw on information from the records and feedback we received relating to the training courses; from participant and non-participant observations made by staff; from records of the ongoing support and training meetings; and from the qualitative interviews (both individual and group) conducted during the course of the project (see Table 6.1). Together, these opportunities and experiences of voluntary work illustrate the extent to which older people can, with appropriate support and encouragement, be enabled to become skilled and effective helpers for members of their peer group. The chapter concludes by briefly examining the impact which involvement in the project had on staff.

Volunteering and older people

Traditionally, volunteering among older people has been couched in terms of civic duty and community service to others. The 'Lady Bountiful' image has been hard to shake off, as has the sense of serving those less fortunate than ourselves. In recent years, certainly since the mid-1980s and the inauguration of the Self Health Care in Old Age Project, volunteering has begun to undergo something of a transformation. Part of the difficulty lies in how we define volunteering. Many large-scale studies include only formal activity where people are involved in voluntary work for a particular organization. This of course leaves aside the vast numbers of people who engage in informal caring, voluntarily, for others. It therefore makes it exceedingly difficult to draw firm conclusions about participation levels (Fischer and Schaffer 1993). However, surveys in the UK and in North America have come to broadly similar conclusions about who volunteers and why. Despite the fact that older people have more free time – or leisure time – by dint of being retired, they are in fact less likely to be involved in voluntary activity than younger groups. In Britain, *The 1991 National Survey of Voluntary Activity* (Lynn and Davis Smith 1991) put the figure at four out of ten people aged 50 to 74 compared with six out of ten people aged 35 to 49. These figures are comparable with research in North America, where 40 per cent of people aged 65 to 74 are volunteers (Independent Sector 1988). However, more recent research shows that since the mid-1980s, cultural, demographic and programmatic improvements have led to a growth in volunteering among most age groups (apart from young people between the ages of 18 and 24), with the largest growth among middle-aged and older people (Chambre 1993). The 1997 *National Survey of Volunteering* (Davis Smith 1998) shows, for example, that the participation rate for 65 to 74 year olds grew from 34 per cent (in 1991) to 45 per cent, while the rate for people aged 75 and over increased from 25 per cent to 35 per cent.

Older women are also more likely to participate than older men: in Britain, nearly 50 per cent of third age women take part in voluntary activities compared with 38 per cent of men (Lynn and Davis Smith 1991). Moreover, those still in paid work, who have higher incomes, who come from higher socio-economic groups, who are well educated and who have access to a car are the most likely to volunteer, while those who are widowed are the least likely to do so (Chambre 1987, 1993; Davis Smith 1992; Knapp *et al.* 1996; Davis Smith 1998). In addition, the most common route into volunteering for older people is through contact with a friend or through membership of a particular organization. The 1990 MORI survey showed that only 2 per cent of volunteers came forward after seeing an advert in the local press, and only 1 per cent after hearing about it on local radio.

Volunteers in the Self Health Care in Old Age Project: who participates and why?

Interestingly, while the data we have about people who became involved as volunteers in the Self Health Care in Old Age Project show some similarities with national trends, there are also important differences. As an example, Table 9.1 provides a profile of the first three cohorts of peer health counsellor/CareLine trainees, and details of the routes through which they first heard about these opportunities.

Women volunteers certainly outnumber men, in this instance by nearly three-to-one. This contrasts markedly with national data which reveal that men and women are equally likely to be volunteers (Davis Smith 1998). While three-quarters of the male volunteers in our project were in their sixties and many were recently retired (most within the previous three years), the age distribution for the women was much broader, with a quarter being in their seventies. Other research (Munday 1991) has suggested a link between involvement in voluntary work and the length of time since a person last held a job, concluding that the best time to interest people in voluntary work is either just before, or just after, the cessation of work. While this appears to hold true for the men in our project, it is not the case for women, many of whom had been retired in excess of five years.

In terms of socio-economic status, we can see from Table 9.1 that just over one half of these volunteers' previous occupations could be classed as non-manual, while two-fifths were manual. The minor differences between men

Table 9.1 Profile of peer health counsellor volunteers

	Women		Men		Totals	
	n	*(%)*	*n*	*(%)*	*n*	*(%)*
Age						
under 50	1	(4)	1	(11)	2	(6)
50–9	7	(30)	–	–	7	(22)
60–9	9	(39)	7	(78)	16	(50)
70 plus	6	(26)	1	(11)	7	(22)
Marital status						
married	16	(70)	7	(78)	23	(72)
widowed	6	(26)	1	(11)	7	(22)
single	1	(4)	–	–	1	(3)
div./septd	–	–	1	(11)	1	(3)
Employment						
manual	9	(39)	4	(44)	13	(41)
non-manual	12	(52)	5	(56)	17	(53)
housewife	2	(9)	–	–	2	(6)
Heard about PHC						
other vol. work	12	(52)	5	(56)	17	(53)
local press	6	(26)	2	(22)	8	(25)
from friend	4	(17)	–	–	4	(13)
local radio	1	(4)	1	(11)	2	(6)
other	–	–	1	(11)	1	(3)
Base n	23	(100)	9	(100)	32	(100)

and women in this respect probably reflect the very high levels of female (skilled manual) employment in this geographical area. In addition, this challenges other research which suggests that people in the higher socio-economic groups are at least twice as likely to take part in voluntary activities (Lynn and Davis Smith 1991; Davis Smith 1998).

We can see that approximately three-quarters of both men and women are married but that again contrary to national figures (Lynn and Davis Smith 1991), a substantial proportion of these volunteers are widowed (particularly the women). Our data show that over half of the volunteers heard about it through their involvement in other voluntary work. Some of this was through other activities that they were involved in associated with the Beth Johnson Foundation, while others were unconnected. 'Hearing through the grapevine' in this way and having a propensity to volunteer appear to be crucial. By contrast though, hearing through a friend, while important for some of the women, was not key. In fact, local press was the next most common route, with a quarter of the volunteers having read about peer health counselling. This demonstrates just how important local press is in this particular geographical area because, nationally, only 2 per cent of older people get involved in volunteering this way (MORI 1990).

These findings raise some important issues about the access routes for older people into volunteering, and the nature of older participants, points to which we shall return in the final chapter. Beyond this, access and participation is also intimately bound up with the motivations of volunteers and with the nature of the voluntary work being offered. We turn to look at this in more detail below.

Volunteer motivation

In terms of volunteer motivation, the latest national surveys (Lynn and Davis Smith 1991; Davis Smith 1998) demonstrate that older volunteers are most likely to have been asked to help (rather than to have offered), usually in response to a particular need in the community. They are also more likely than other age groups to have volunteered in order to meet people, to make friends, and because they have time to spare. While our data are not strictly comparable with the quantitative findings from these kinds of studies, identifying and understanding the motivating forces which prompt individuals to volunteer, is vitally important to the work of the Foundation as a whole, and the Self Health Care in Old Age Project in particular. Knowing what motivates people and what they want from their involvement helps us to recognize the needs of volunteers, plan appropriate training and support, and explore what can be offered in terms of the available choices.

Motivation was therefore key, and uncovered at various points in the recruitment and training process through both formal and informal means. Chapter 5 noted that people who responded to the recruitment drives for peer health counselling volunteers were all put through an initial selection process, completing a detailed form, providing two references and undergoing an interview. The form includes an open-ended question asking what it is that particularly interests the individual in the Peer Health Counselling scheme, while part of the subsequent interview also explores how committed and motivated people are for voluntary work and whether they are willing and able to learn (Ivers and Meade 1991). Once on the training course, issues about motivation, why people are there and what they hope to gain from it, come through very strongly. Similarly, older people who volunteer to take part in other aspects of the Foundation's work are also required to undergo a selection and training process.

Experience over many years has led us to identify a range of motivations for older people undertaking voluntary work. Many of these, while still resonating with the traditional association about providing a service to others and of helping those perhaps 'less fortunate' than ourselves, are very much about meeting the needs of older people for satisfying and challenging opportunities in retirement. These motivations are by no means mutually exclusive and it is important to note that some, or indeed all of them, can apply at different points in the lives of volunteers. The motivations of volunteers in the Peer Health Counselling scheme are also not unique to that project, and similar reasons are expressed by volunteers in other parts of the programme, whether they be running CareLine, serving in the Health Shop or perhaps leading a group of ramblers or swimmers. In no priority order, our older volunteers volunteer in order to:

- *Help others* – This was a very common motivation, but one with caveats attached to it in the sense that people talked about 'helping people of my own age', and of wanting to help other people 'to feel as well, and be as healthy as, me'. In other words, it was primarily about mutual help and support and about extending the abilities of those 'natural helpers' who had been identified very early on in the development of the project (see Chapter 5).
- *Feel useful and valued* – This appears from our work to be the overriding motivation. Many of the people with whom we have had contact through the project feel strongly that they are marginalized and are considered as no longer contributing to society. Particularly where they have recently retired from paid work, they talk in terms of loss of confidence and feeling redundant. Voluntary work offers one way, they feel, of helping regain a positive self-image and building self-confidence.
- *Make friends and combat loneliness* – Leaving work, perhaps before one's husband or partner does, together with bereavement, can dramatically alter people's social networks and opportunities for social contact especially if these have not been very well developed earlier in life. A great number of the older volunteers with whom we have worked see volunteering as a way of reaching out, both to re-engage and to make new friendships. We saw the importance of this in Chapter 8 when discussing participation in the LAY courses, and this reason is as true for volunteering as for participation.
- *Give structure and purpose to the day* – While older volunteers certainly seem to have more spare time as other research suggests, the crucial dimension for our volunteers concerned the need to have a framework to what they were doing: a framework which for many was previously supplied by the routines associated with paid work even when that work, as it was for a lot of the women, was part-time.

- *Utilize existing skills* – This too was very important to older people many of whom had acquired a lifetime of experiences and skills which they were keen to pass on to others. In the context of the Peer Health Counselling project, this revolved around a variety of sports and health-related activities, skills from previous voluntary work, and skills from their paid work and from domestic contexts.
- *Learn, and pass on, new skills* – For many, an additional motivation was the chance to develop new skills, especially if they had been channelled earlier on in life into a job or career path which had given them very little opportunity to explore other avenues. Many felt it would open up new horizons for them and offer them challenging and exciting interests.
- *To enjoy themselves* – With time on their hands, and desires to perhaps make new friends, combat loneliness and structure their days, as well as to use existing skills or learn new ones, an additional motivation was seeing volunteering as an enjoyable and rewarding activity in, and of, itself.

The needs and motivations of volunteers are therefore as important as the needs of the project, and there has to be a reciprocal relationship between the two. It is no use for instance, to put a volunteer into a setting which will damage, rather than enhance, their self-confidence and self-esteem. Consequently, 'matching' volunteer needs to particular areas of work within the project was key, as was the opportunity for people to move on to different and/or additional areas of work as they developed and should they express a wish to. To illustrate these issues concerning access routes, needs and motivations, let us now consider the experiences of a number of our volunteers.

Access: pathways into volunteering

Research findings suggest that volunteering in later life tends to be built on a lifetime of volunteer involvement (Chambre 1987; Davis Smith 1992). For many of the volunteers in the project, this was indeed the case. Eleanor Wainwright, now a peer health counsellor, said: 'I've always been a volunteer – right from the age of say 33 or 34, when I joined the Civil Defence as it was then – from Civil Defence to St John Ambulance'. Maud Jones, a CareLine volunteer, recalled: 'I started as a volunteer many years ago with the WRVS delivering meals-on-wheels'.

Arthur Machin took early retirement at the age of 61 after 30 years with the same firm. He was doing voluntary work with his old company, visiting retired workers, when this happened to him:

> I was driving around in my car when I heard on the radio that Beth Johnson wanted some volunteers to organise a booklet about the various clubs in the area. So I thought, 'This is something I'll have a go at'. Four of us turned up. We each took a section of the Stoke-on-Trent area and got together a valuable booklet which told us where all the clubs were and what they did.

From this, Arthur got involved with the establishment of the Leisure Association in 1982 and has been integral to its development ever since. When asked about his motivations for engaging in voluntary work, he commented:

It means to me that instead of just getting up every morning and thinking, 'What have I got to do now?', or 'What shall we do?', I know exactly how my day is planned. I know where I'm going to go and what I'm going to do, and what pleasure I'm going to give to the people when I get there. And I think when you do retire, you haven't got to just sit about and watch the TV all day long. You've got to motivate yourself in finding something to do. And I think if you do this, and keep yourself reasonably fit, you're going a long way to enjoy your retirement for one thing!

For Arthur, his motivations for volunteering have included keeping himself occupied, helping and encouraging others, and getting enjoyment and pleasure out of what he is doing.

We can contrast these lifelong volunteers who now work as peer health counsellors and activities' leaders with others for whom volunteering was a new departure.

Fred Evans was aged 60 when he was interviewed, and had been a volunteer at the Senior Centre since the early days of its existence. The youngest of six children (four boys and two girls), he left school at the age of 14 and went to work in a porcelain factory where one of his sisters was also employed. Apart from two years in the forces, Fred worked at the same place until, at the age of 50, he was made redundant. Having never married and having lived with his widowed mother (his father died when Fred was a teenager), Fred found his changed circumstances difficult to cope with:

I didn't want to leave, but the firm went into liquidation. We were told one day that the firm had closed, and not to return. There was no chance of other jobs and we were signing on at the dole, and calling in the labour exchange. I didn't make any preparation for retirement. I had depression following the redundancy . . . and mother died two and a half years after my redundancy.

Quite by chance, Fred called in one day at the Senior Centre for a cup of tea, got talking, and has not looked back since. He helps out with general tasks in and around the centre and in the kitchen. His initial motivation for becoming involved in voluntary work was largely about combating his depression and isolation. It was also a means of providing him with social contact and friendship as well as about giving form and structure to his day.

Dora Chaney retired at the age of 60 after a lifetime's work as a cook in school and factory canteens. Twice married, widowed, and with seven adult children whose ages span 20 years, she discovered voluntary work after the death of her second husband. She describes her motivation and experience of becoming involved in a very matter-of-fact way:

After my husband died, I was sitting about at home and thought 'Well, what do I do now? I've got a big family, but they're out at work all day'. I thought, I just can't sit here and vegetate. So one day, I went to the centre – as a customer – and they gave me a cup of tea which they said is 'on the house', and this lady came and talked with me . . . and eventually she asked me if I'd be interested in voluntary work. So I said, 'Oh yes I would'. So from then on, I've done the voluntary work.

Moreover, as we shall see later in this chapter, Dora has expanded her voluntary activities from using her culinary skills in the kitchen to peer health counselling work in a variety of settings.

Jean Marson also became involved in voluntary work through the Senior Centre. Jean had been born and brought up in the local area although, as a child, she moved around quite a lot: 'we moved from one rented house to another quite frequently. We moved because she [her mother] liked living in different houses. It meant I had to get used to different schools'. Her father was a self-employed barber and her mother took in lodgers and, at the age of 14, she herself started work as an apprentice paintress. At 16 she went to work as a chambermaid in one of the big hotels and at 18 she married a cobbler. Later in their married life, he too went into the pottery industry though she never returned to work 'apart for a little – about three years – when my son went to school because we wanted the extra money. Since then I've just had little jobs'.

Having travelled the familiar road of job, marriage, children and part-time work, Jean found herself, at the age of 61, with time on her hands, and a husband who was still working long hours and was not due to retire for another six months. She describes her route into the project, and what she subsequently did, in these words:

> I first heard about the Beth Johnson Foundation when you were at St John's church [the first location for the Senior Centre]. I got in with this lady and became friendly, and she said 'Why don't you come in with us, and help us, and be with us?' I did work in the kitchen, and serving in the Senior Centre . . . it fills quite a big gap in my day and the reason I came was for somewhere to go.

For Jean, the prime motivations were concerned with occupying her time and giving her somewhere to go and, having started out as a volunteer in the Senior Centre, she then moved into the shop.

Like Jean, *Edwina Clayton* came from a local working-class family. As one of five children, with a mother who did not work 'because of having a large family', and a father who 'did a lot of different jobs mainly because of unemployment at that time', she grew up 'aware of the hardship'. Although Edwina felt that her parents would have liked her to have a more thorough education and she 'loved school', she had to leave at 14 because 'the finance wasn't there'. Her eldest brother passed the examinations to go to the high school and got a scholarship, but her parents could not afford for the other children to stay on. Looking back, Edwina said:

> I don't think I realized then that education was so important . . . Had things been different I would possibly have gone onto higher education, but my mother was pleased I got a job. You were lucky if you could get a job then. I didn't regret leaving school, because that was what you had to do then.

Her first job was as a shop assistant where she stayed until the Second World War started when she was 19. She then went into the Women's Auxiliary Air Force for three years learning, much to her surprise, to be a flight mechanic ('I wasn't mechanically minded!') and then a switchboard operator. During the war, she married a local boy and after she and her husband were demobbed, she went back to work as a shop assistant. Throughout her adult life she worked part-time at this and, at other times, as a clerk and as a switchboard operator while she brought up her two daughters. She retired at the age of 60 but said:

> I retired at 60 and didn't want to leave. The times I lived in, there wasn't really an awareness of retirement. When you have worked all those years from 14 to 60 – apart from two years – I quite looked forward to it . . . but at first, I was very unsettled. I felt that at first it was abrupt. I think your employment could have gradually retired you so that it wasn't such a shock. There was no schemes where you did half . . . One week you are fully occupied as a worker and finish on a Saturday, and on Monday there is no work . . . I was dissatisfied, perhaps I was a bit discontented. Personally, I had no income of my own; I didn't have my own money; there was no routine in my life, and I missed my social life and the company, having worked with a lot of people. That is suddenly shut off.

Then, one day, this happened to her:

> I was going to Hanley on the bus, and I often get talking to someone on the bus. She was saying that she always goes into the shop on a Friday to have some lunch. And I said, 'Which shop did she mean?' She said, 'The Beth Johnson Shop' . . . she said she goes and there's leaflets for the elderly, and things that you could do. I didn't go in, but thought I would go next time.
>
> I went into the shop the next time and Betty [the Health Shop manager] was there, and I think Pauline [the volunteer support and training officer] was there. I looked at the leaflets and there was also a notice up for someone for CareLine. I spoke to Betty about it and she took my name and address and asked if I could supply two references, which I did . . . I started on a Monday and I still do Mondays.

A chance meeting on a bus triggered off the chain of events that led to Edwina fulfilling her need to be 'a help to older people'. Her practical skills as a switchboard operator, combined with her interpersonal skills from years as a shop assistant, have found an outlet in her work as a peer health counsellor working on CareLine. This has helped her to replace the social circle she badly missed when she had to retire, makes her feel useful and valued, has boosted her confidence and opened up new avenues for her as she ventures into other activities within the project.

Joyce Randall too came into the project in the wake of being bereaved. She recalled:

> I heard it on the radio while I was sitting knitting. I thought it was something I could do [volunteering] so I finished the row, went straight out and got a bus to Hanley. I've been with the project ever since.

Like Edwina, Joyce began work in the shop, preparing and serving food and, while she used her cooking skills to invent new recipes, she has also gone on to work on CareLine.

For many of these people, and indeed others involved with the Self Health Care in Old Age Project, becoming a volunteer often represented the start of a new phase in their lives, even if they had been a volunteer previously. Other choices also opened up to them as they took up opportunities to enhance existing skills and learn new ones.

The challenges of voluntary work

Conventionally, studies of volunteering suggest that the most common activities among older volunteers are raising or handling money, helping to organize or run events, serving on committees and visiting other elderly people (Davis Smith 1992). However, the academic research also shows that they are much less likely than younger groups to see volunteering as an opportunity to learn new skills (Davis Smith 1998). While the Foundation's volunteers certainly engage in some of these activities, our experience in the Self Health Care in Old Age Project draws attention to the need to move away from traditional, welfarist approaches and simplistic notions of altruistic service to others and consider what makes for challenging and stimulating voluntary activity, what volunteers learn as well as offer, and how the development of new skills can be encouraged and supported.

Choosing what to do

As a prelude to this, however, it is important that potential volunteers have a sense of what they are being asked to undertake and that they are enabled to make informed choices about the kinds of activities they are most suited for. This process begins, as we noted in Chapter 5, with recruitment and training. Talking about the initial training, John Brown (who eventually went on to lead groups of older people in health-related activities) encapsulates many of the anxieties, doubts and uncertainties people have at this time:

> It has made me think, 'Am I capable of putting this over to other people?' That's my doubt. I don't quite know. This is all fascinating to me but, I think, 'Have I got the confidence to put this over to other people?' That's my doubt at the moment.

Others too express concerns about the kinds of voluntary work they might undertake. Jean Marson for example was adamant about not getting involved in work with groups: 'Not groups. I don't think I could cope with groups'. This was in sharp contrast to Dora Chaney who spoke enthusiastically about how she might like to undertake this kind of work:

> I would like to get in with elderly people because I think if you get a group together it's surprising how much you can learn from them. I think they need to get together to get them out of themselves . . . and if you talk about what you did in your lifetime, then somebody else may think that they want to as well. It's surprising what they can learn about each other.

However, with further training and support at monthly meetings, volunteers visibly grow in confidence and most find that their skills develop and their participation is something they come to value greatly and enjoy. As Marjory Simpson, now a peer health counsellor, observed: 'Before I came here I thought, "Oh no, you're not going to get me on this lark". Yet now I feel at home and think, "Yes, I could do this".' Similarly, Joyce Randall, remembered how the training was 'great fun, and gave me confidence ready for the real thing'. Edwina Clayton, talking about the training and her work on CareLine, noted: 'I thought CareLine was originally just being a telephonist. The training made me realize the importance of listening carefully and I now know that having a smile in your voice is most necessary if calling housebound and depressed people.'

So, in addition to initial training being important for enabling people to make informed choices about what they wished to do, it also begins the process of skills development – whether that be awakening old skills or learning new ones.

Sharing, developing and learning new skills

Each of the volunteers we have already met describes, in interview, how they have become better informed and what skills they have learnt through both the training and the actual voluntary work they have undertaken. With respect to the training, the evaluation forms they completed (see Table 6.1) indicate how they learnt particular factual things linked with the three main themes: ageing and ageism, positive health in old age, and helping relationships. They now feel they are able to:

- think constructively about some of the problems associated with old age;
- see how stereotypes get developed and reinforced and what impact ageist views have on them as individuals and on older people more generally;
- understand the different components which go into developing and maintaining good health;
- think about how change affects them as individuals and how they can help others to change and modify their habits and lifestyles;
- be more confident in their dealings with others;
- be good listeners;
- understand, learn and use stress management and relaxation techniques for their own, and others' benefit;
- access and use information and resources.

In interview, Dora Chaney remembered how she 'found all the talks so interesting, and I really listened. We have learned some entirely new things and built up some confidence.' In similar vein, Marjory Simpson recalled: 'I found that I was beginning to lose confidence in myself, and being able to listen to other people talk, and being able to say some of the things that I have remembered or recalled, has given me added confidence.'

John Brown noted:

> There were so many new aspects that I've wondered about, and never really got down to doing . . . I think the other thing is the depth of thinking that this has provoked . . . I feel that most of us have had cause to

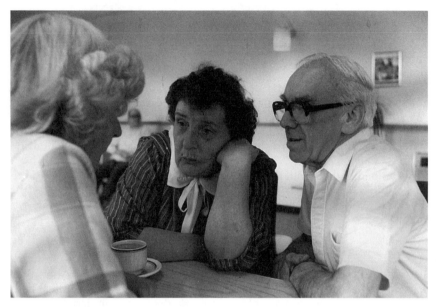

Personal counselling

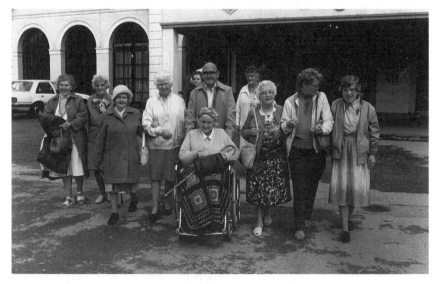

CareLine volunteers and clients go out for the day

think much more deeply about many things – more than we would have dreamed of – and having tasted it, you want some more.

Beyond the passing on of factual information, and the stimulation to think more deeply about things, a further key feature of the induction training has been the emphasis on sharing particular skills and interests. On the first courses, these extracurricular activities were chalked up on a blackboard and fitted in around the programmed sessions. However, as the value of this became increasingly apparent, special time was set aside on subsequent courses for the sharing of these activities and skills, either through practical demonstrations, or through getting members of the group to prepare short talks about their hobbies or interests. Staff too took a full part in these activities.

The importance of this lies in enabling volunteers and staff to learn more about each other and to value the interests and life experiences of everyone in the group. While many volunteers again were initially anxious about this aspect, speaking and/or demonstrating in front of their peers was for many a confidence booster, and a recognition and affirmation that they indeed had skills to contribute. In fact, the real skill was in getting people to stop, once they had started!

As Cyril Walker observed: 'I think that adding to the programme all the extra curricular activities, made it marvellous. All of us had something to give, and you have a great sense of exchange.'

John Brown endorsed this view:

The very act of sharing an activity makes you very close to the person. We are doing things with other people. People are being open to the experience and saying, 'Yes, I'll try it'. I had this personal experience when Roy came running with me, never having done it before. It was the same with the music at lunch time, and with the meditation. We didn't do it in order to find companions, we did it in order to do the activity. Sharing the activity makes a sort of bond.

Dora Chaney noted how much they got from being prepared to share skills and interests with each other:

The way that people did come and share with others, and people received whatever the other person's skill was, and they seriously contemplated what was being offered. That was probably the most rewarding thing for me, because people were seriously applying themselves to what other people had to offer, which doesn't always happen does it? Sometimes people just say that it's wonderful, but they don't try to join in with the skill of the other person.

Beyond this, ongoing skills development has been a vital ingredient of the whole project. As noted in Chapter 5, support and training are continuous features. At regular monthly meetings organized by the support worker, volunteers kept up to date with what each other was doing, sharing successes and discussing any difficulties that may have arisen. Newer volunteers derived benefit from the experiences of the old hands and, in addition, there were opportunities for further training around specific issues and for considering ideas for new avenues of work.

The monthly topics undertaken included, for example, sessions on what the body is capable of doing; incontinence; exercise and diet; diabetes; nutrition; and counselling techniques. These were interspersed with in-depth discussion about the day-to-day work that people were doing; with arranged half-day visits for volunteers to observe others at work (in residential homes, health clinics, pensioners' clubs, day centres and schools); and with small group exercises around the practical considerations and hurdles to developing work in other settings (for example, stimulating activity in a residential home; undertaking reminiscence work; or running an information and advice stall in a health centre). The aim of these sessions was to build on the understanding, knowledge and skills that people had and, again, to help volunteers find their most appropriate niche in the project.

As the Self Health Care in Old Age Project developed, volunteers from other parts of the Foundation's work were incorporated into this wider support and training network. This enabled some to move into other areas of voluntary work in the project which they might previously have felt were not for them, as well as opening up the opportunity to enhance old skills or learn new ones. For Jean Marson, whom we met earlier, working as a volunteer in the Senior Health Shop, preparing and serving food, proved informative in a number of ways. She suffers with diabetes but said:

> I think I have learned quite a bit about health by working in the shop. I have to be careful with my diet, and I have made a few changes in the things I eat. Coming here, rather than a health centre, I feel you are able to talk more freely: it's easier and you get quite a lot of advice here.

She mentioned how much she enjoyed working with other volunteers, and about the confidence it had given her: 'I think I would be able to find out about help available if I became dependent. I wouldn't mind asking for help if I needed it now'. Interestingly, these observations are very close to some of the comments made by shop customers in Chapter 7.

Dora Chaney, having begun by cooking and serving meals in the Senior Centre, became a peer health counsellor. Dora undertook the training and, in addition to her work at the centre, was one of the band of volunteers who went out to undertake group work in various institutional settings, leading gentle exercise sessions and health discussion groups. Like all peer health counsellors, she filled in weekly records of her activities and then brought them to the monthly support meetings. These records document her work in residential homes and sheltered housing and show that in these settings, and in the Senior Centre, she was also engaged in one-to-one discussions with people about their health, often around issues to do with taking up new activities and/or about physical activity and exercise. She recorded that 'helping people feel at ease' and 'answering specific questions' were activities she was often engaged in. Some of the written comments on her record sheets expand on these activities:

> On Wednesday, I did some counselling with two ladies – both at different times. The first lady came to see what we do at the centre. She had retired, but her husband still went to work and she said that she would

come again and bring friends with her. The other lady, I am happy to report, has now joined our art class.

Discussed with the residents ways in which we, as peer health counsellors, could help improve mobility, self-help, diet etc.

The class [in a residential home] continues to be popular with the staff and the residents, and there are definite signs of improvement in the movement of limbs of some of the residents . . . We set up an information table with leaflets, and the residents were very interested in these.

I talked this week on Thursday with a nice couple. They had both retired and needed some activity they could do together. I first told them about our dancing and about rambling, and am happy to report they have taken up the dancing.

In interview, Dora feels that, in addition to the skills she already possessed, she has undoubtedly learnt new skills, especially in the areas of communication and listening, and in leading gentle exercise and discussion groups. She comments:

I go to old people's homes and we do exercises to music with them. Now, before I joined the peer health counsellors, no way would I have thought of doing anything like that. But now, having learnt it from the Beth Johnson Foundation, I could go and do it myself.

Other volunteers like Fred Evans, while they may not have found additional outlets for their skills, have continued to learn. Fred has stayed with the Senior Centre for many years now, and has learnt about staying healthy in old age. He has talked with others at the centre – both volunteers and participants – and has observed the health-related classes and activities, saying 'I am level headed about food now . . . and I have a reasonable diet and take a reasonable amount of exercise'. These comments echo those from some of the participants in the Look After Yourself courses (see Chapter 8).

These examples illustrate some of the ways in which skills enhancement and development are integrally linked with participation. In this sense, participation extends beyond just the facts and figures of who is involved, and reaches out to incorporate what it is these volunteers actually do and, most importantly, what they gain from their participation.

Beyond participation

Research on volunteering among older people shows that once they become involved they in fact give more time to volunteering than younger people. The 1991 National Survey found, for example, that volunteers aged 65 to 74 spent an average of five hours per week on their voluntary activities compared with an average of less than three hours for all other groups (Lynn and Davis Smith 1991). In the United States, older volunteers give an average six hours per week compared with three and a half for other adults (Independent Sector 1988). They also bring considerable benefits to organizations in that they stay longer (four out of ten third age volunteers have been involved with the same organization for ten years or more, compared with only two in ten volunteers aged 35 to 49) and have a fund of skills and experience (Butler and Gleason 1985; Dychtwald and Flower 1989; Lynn and Davis Smith 1991; Newman *et al.* 1997). In this sense, they represent a rich resource and a good 'investment' in terms of funds which might be spent on training and support (Ellis and Noyes 1990; Davis Smith 1992).

Volunteers in the Self Health Care in Old Age Project certainly bear out these points. More than a decade after it began, many volunteers still work with the Foundation. A small-scale study of one of the CareLines found that out of the six women interviewed, five had been operating the line for five years or more (Deakin 1998). Moreover, four of them gave between four and ten hours per week to their voluntary activities and, although restricted through lack of education and (in some instances) poor health, they were very committed to this work, often combining it with other more informal voluntary activities. A particular advantage of working on the CareLine was that the time commitment was very clear although the work itself was often emotionally demanding. Fran and Elaine, two of the volunteers, articulated it in these terms:

> Only a minimum amount of time was required. Knowing the timescale that they were expecting and the level of commitment was good because I had got time to think out my home situation . . . which was better than enthusiastically volunteering for something where you're not quite sure what the level of commitment is and then having to say, 'No, I am sorry, I can't do this'. [Fran]

> I love being with people and meeting people, and I think as you get older, while you still have a lot to give, you really don't want to be too committed. With this job, you can give all that you can to the client but, when you've finished on the telephone, that's it. There is no more commitment. That's what I particularly like. [Elaine]
>
> (Deakin 1998: 33)

Like the other volunteers we have heard from above, these women also value the ongoing support and training, noting how useful and necessary it is for, without it, 'you wouldn't hold the team together' [Elaine]. The meetings also enable them to 'share your feelings and upsets with others who understand and share the experiences' [Fran] (Deakin 1998: 34).

By way of contrast, some of the other peer health counsellors (and indeed, activities' leaders) participated for inordinate amounts of time. The weekly record sheets reveal some volunteers engaging in this work on every day of the week – Saturdays and Sundays included. Evidently, for a small number of volunteers, their participation has gone beyond a circumscribed, fixed time commitment, to become a way of life. Jane Brownsword, for example, from one of the early groups of trainee peer health counsellors, indicated how, during a typical week, she would participate in the following:

> Saturday, Sunday and Monday – at home, but working on a one-to-one basis talking to individuals, answering specific questions, discussing general health and well-being, and helping a lady get her husband to hospital after he had had a stroke.

Tuesday – in a residential home or a sheltered housing complex, working with a group, leading gentle exercise and discussion of health and well-being.

Wednesday, Thursday, Friday – in the Senior Centre, working on a one-to-one basis (Wed and Fri) and with a group (Wed and Thurs), helping people feel at ease, discussing health and well-being, answering specific questions and advising people.

More commonly though, both peer health counsellors and CareLine volunteers would participate on either one or two days per week, giving their time exceedingly regularly week-in, week-out.

Volunteering as empowerment

Finally then, in our consideration of the impact of this work on volunteers, we have to ask what was it they gained from their involvement? We have seen that many of them rediscovered old skills, learnt new things, became more aware of their own and others' health needs, gained in confidence, found companionship, fulfilment and enjoyment in their voluntary work. Again, as with the shop customers (see Chapter 7) and the LAY participants (see Chapter 8) these are clear signs of empowerment and further illustration of the incremental and complex processes by which health promotion is achieved and then maintained. Although none of those whom we observed or spoke to in interview situations over the years talked specifically in terms of empowerment, the rewards and benefits that they gained are evident in the things they do and say about the impact of volunteering on their lives.

Fred Evans, our Senior Centre volunteer, although still suffering with bouts of depression, said this about his involvement:

It takes you away from four walls. Home is nothing if there's nobody there. Although I see the neighbours every day, and my brothers are nearby and there's no reason for me not to go visiting every day, it isn't how I want it – only going from one house to another . . . I have seen it [the Senior Centre] develop. It's done me good all round knowing that such a thing is going . . . I've learnt to get a satisfied mind and sociability – togetherness . . . I'm attracted to the routine. I should miss it if I couldn't come. I'm a stayer . . . I would rather come here than go to the pub.

For Fred, volunteering seems to have provided him with a source of contentment in addition to the sociability aspect we noted earlier. From this, he has gone on to develop a sense of feeling useful and a valued part of the development of the centre.

Dora Chaney talked at some length about her volunteer involvement, about the anxieties of the early days, and about what it meant to her:

I did feel frightened going in for the first day – rather nervous. But once I got through the door it was great. There was such a welcome then and I thought, 'This is definitely something I can do from now until I'm too old' . . . I've never looked back since, I really enjoy it: there's something for me to go out to every day.

Her confidence has developed to such an extent that, with the knowledge she has acquired, she feels that she could now set up projects similar to the Senior Centre: 'I could now. Before this, no. But now I could run a centre on me own along similar lines. I've learnt from the Foundation how it's done. I could do it – organize classes etcetera . . . I could do it now with a good set of volunteers'. Dora has widened her repertoire of skills considerably to take in not only her kitchen work but also group and individual peer health counselling activities.

Similarly, *Jean Marson*, having started out in the Senior Centre, developed the confidence to move into the shop, while *Joyce Randall* recalled how her involvement with CareLine enabled her to overcome her bereavement and move on:

> I've just moved into the shop from the Senior Centre. I do Wednesday, Thursday and Friday because my husband does long hours . . . I find it very interesting to meet people who are coming in and I get to know a lot of the customers. [Jean]

> I enjoy all the contacts and I get satisfaction from assisting the customers, and relief from sharing experiences with other volunteers and staff. I learn from them and I teach them my skills. I get a lot of satisfaction from it and I have since become a Macmillan volunteer too. It was so hard for me without any help, and I hope I can offer others a little help now. The project is great – there's nowhere else like it. [Joyce]

Edwina Clayton and *Arthur Machin* summed up what, for many of the volunteers, it was all about:

> it gives you a purpose in life when you're retired. It is a new way of life . . . I enjoy thinking that in a way I am being a help to older people. You get an interest in the way they talk to you and their problems . . . you are helping in a small way. It is something you can give . . . you can get in a group of people the same age, you get the confidence to think 'this is good, this is important' . . . they are giving each other the confidence. [Edwina]

> We're of an age now when you can find other things more interesting than what it was going into work. And now I don't know how I found time to go to work . . . it's a grand life, this time you're not at work. [Arthur]

The impact on staff

Finally we briefly consider how the project impacted on the paid staff. Again, we have to be selective in the issues and illustrations we can include here. Consequently, we shall focus on the interaction between the action and research elements of the project in an effort to demonstrate how staff learnt to integrate the two, as well as sharing and acquiring skills.

It will be recalled from Chapter 6 that we wanted the project to reflect and resonate with the kinds of change-oriented and empowering action research now increasingly being written about in the academic literature (Reinharz 1992; Hart and Bond 1995). However, there is always a danger in any project such as this that because the project developers and the researchers are so closely intertwined, that we perhaps see change where in reality there is none. In other words, we are so invested in making the project a success that it blinds us to a more critical or objective evaluation of what has transpired. We adopted a number of strategies to try to minimize this danger.

First, the three core staff responsible for the development of the project had, at one level, clearly defined roles: as project officer, as project director/promoter and as project evaluator. As these titles suggest, the project officer was primarily responsible for the day-to-day running of the four elements of the project and for the line management of staff employed through the project (whether project funded or financed through other sources). Overall control of the project was the director's responsibility, including financial management and liaison with funding bodies. Monitoring and evaluation was the main function of the project evaluator. This formal division of roles and responsibilities, while important, probably belies the extent of close interaction and overlap which in fact occurred between people on a day-to-day basis. As is common within many small voluntary agencies, people have in effect to work very closely together and sometimes substitute for one another. We were though able to establish a relationship such that the project officer came to view the evaluator as 'like my shadow', while the director describes the symbiotic relationship between research, developments and policy in these terms:

> Our researcher helps projects establish monitoring procedures and reviews them regularly, with project staff, to see what lessons can be learned. She is also part of the Foundation influencing and moulding policy, and a part of the management team, making decisions about finance and examining what is happening by field work at the grass roots. At the same time she is able to withdraw from all this when necessary and report to us on the Foundation's work with a long-term view. It means a shift from one role to the other, but she can do it because of her academic training. She will never compromise her academic integrity. When we have shifted from our objectives, she tells us.
>
> (Ball 1988: 18)

Second, we engaged in as much (recorded) discussion as possible throughout the duration of the project, attempting to involve staff and volunteers at all stages, in the choice, design, piloting and administration of the selected methods, as well as in the emerging analyses. Following each data collection exercise at, for example, the quarterly censuses in the Health Shop, the project evaluator would carry out a very quick, preliminary analysis of the material producing a short discussion document divided into two columns: 'Findings' and 'Issues for discussion and action'. These documents were circulated and, within a fortnight, a (tape-recorded) meeting would be held to review the material. The ensuing minutes and action plans would then be widely circulated and discussed further within the project.

Third, as observed in Chapter 6, external evaluation procedures were in place under the auspices of the European Commission's Animation and Dissemination Service. This meant that help was available outside the immediate project should it be required. In these ways, we attempted to balance the action and research elements, all the time learning as we went along, what an appropriate balance might be at any given time. This balance tended to alter over the course of the project as we became more skilled and confident with what we were doing in both research and development terms. For example, in the very early stages of the project, our external evaluator commented that:

> I was impressed by what I saw – namely three individuals working very closely together as a team with very complementary skills, entrepreneurial in outlook, and with a firm commitment to the principles of community development and handing over initiatives to volunteer groups as soon as possible.
>
> (Letter and report, 7 April 1986)

As we continued to develop the project and our monitoring and evaluation procedures, we had less recourse to the Animation and Dissemination Service. The major challenge for us as staff became not only about our ability to work together as a team, but also to effect some real development and change for us as individuals, and also for the rest of the staff and volunteers associated with the project.

Drawing on information contained in various reports and analyses, we can present snapshots of some of these changes. For example, less than a year into the project, the project officer made the following pertinent observations on some of the issues raised above:

> Our project is monitored continuously by the Foundation's research officer and all staff are involved in discussions before and after our quarterly census weeks. It is not always easy to allocate the necessary time to this discussion, especially for staff who operate essentially at field work level.
>
> Similarly, the analysis of research material, which takes place during discussions, requires us all to make objective observations about our daily work – a process more familiar to researchers than to community workers who, of necessity, become closely involved in the daily round and relationships.
>
> We are all learning from the process and, after two census weeks and four meetings, I feel that we are all beginning to understand better the benefits of this dual approach to a new initiative and to appreciate the differing, though complementary role of each member of the team.
>
> (Report, June 1987)

Other staff noticed developments and changes in themselves and others. For example, the administrative assistant in the shop expanded her role considerably, becoming particularly interested in supporting the volunteers. The project officer reported how this individual was 'visibly developing and expanding her horizons' (Report, June 1987) and, when we held a long review meeting half-way through the project, the administrative assistant herself talked about how satisfied she was that she was 'able to help people and be useful'. These comments, and similar ones from the volunteer support and training officer about how pleased she was at 'being wanted', echo quite closely some of the gains identified by the volunteers themselves.

Finally, it was evident that the staff team as a whole became much more research minded and research aware over the duration of the project. The monitoring and evaluation of the project was set up, as we have seen, to be a combined effort between the staff, the volunteers and the research officer. Underlying this was a belief that research could and should become an integral part of people's day-to-day work. This became a reality when I moved to Keele University midway through the initial funding period. While I retained oversight of the evaluation, staff and volunteers themselves felt sufficiently skilled and able to continue to monitor the various elements of the project using the previously developed tools.

Conclusion

The experience of the Self Health Care in Old Age Project (as well as subsequent developments) provides many lessons for the Foundation and for other organizations and agencies who strive to work with older people. These lessons will be considered in the final chapter but for now, I hope that readers will indulge me while I close this present discussion with a brief personal observation about what my own involvement in the project meant to me.

I am privileged to have worked as the Foundation's research officer between 1982 and 1988 and to have retained my involvement with the organization, first through a continuation of the project, then as a member of one of its main committees and, latterly, as the member of the advisory group for the Foundation's Intergenerational Programme with particular responsibility for research support and advice. It was during my time at the Foundation – and specifically in connection with the Self Health Care in Old Age Project – that I undoubtedly learnt my craft as a social researcher. It was possible for me, during this time, to learn about and experience first-hand very many aspects associated with action research and to have close and regular interaction with older people. This is a luxury rarely afforded to conventional academic researchers. Moreover, as has been noted with volunteers and with project participants, it was the fundamental belief and trust shown in me by my colleagues that was key to my own development and growing skills and confidence as a social gerontologist – to my own sense of empowerment.

10

Learning the lessons: the role of self health care in future policy and practice

Introduction

This final chapter draws together the findings from the Self Health Care in Old Age Project with the analyses of the theoretical and conceptual elements in the first half of the book. The major contention of this chapter – and indeed of the entire book – is that while much has been done, it is still very piecemeal and fragmented. We urgently need to draw together the elements of best practice in this arena, in order to shape and inform health policy around this issue. Innovative projects are all well and good but unless they are properly researched and evaluated and the findings fed into wider debates and discussions, they will simply remain as localized examples. The primary purpose of this chapter therefore is to consider the main lessons which we need to learn. We begin this process by summarizing and critically reflecting on our key findings before moving on to look at lessons for practice, and associated lessons for policy.

The Self Health Care in Old Age Project: success or failure?

Answering such a question categorically is, of course, notoriously difficult and the most accurate response is probably 'successful in parts'. It is also important to bear in mind that much of the data presented in Chapters 7–9 have come from participants in the project as opposed to non-participants. Our research resources did not extend to following up people who, for whatever reason, may have dropped out at various points. Crucially then, one might argue that an overly rosy picture has been presented. Thus, an additional aim of this chapter is to begin the task of thinking a little more critically about what success or failure might mean for projects such as our own, and what lessons this holds for wider health promotion policy and practice with older people. Importantly too, we should remind ourselves at the start of this summary that the project was also externally evaluated and many of its positive impacts endorsed through this process (Greengross and Batty 1989; Room 1990). However, what is also clear is that some aspects of the project have worked out better than others. In order to consider these issues in more detail, we return to the aims of the project and, in particular, to the main criteria of *participation, accessibility, informed choice, skills development* and *empowerment* against which we have been evaluating the various activities. Figure 10.1 shows these dimensions diagrammatically.

Who participates?

Looking at the project in action, it is evident that in terms of *participation*, considerable numbers of older people have come into contact with its four main elements: the Senior Health Shop, peer health counselling, CareLine and health-related activities. We saw in Chapter 7 that literally thousands of older people have been through the doors of the Senior Health Shop, partaking of refreshments, collecting leaflets, hearing talks about various aspects of health in old age, being weighed or having their blood pressure taken, and talking with staff and peer health counsellors about issues of concern. Many older people too have found their way to the Senior Centre to participate in activities ranging from dancing to yoga to painting to keep fit. Specific courses – notably the Look After Yourself ones – have proved a vital and enduring feature of this approach. In Chapter 8, we learnt how the participants of these early courses were sufficiently motivated to continue with them even in the absence of a tutor, and how demand has meant that two courses now run regularly one after another throughout the year. Beyond these courses, and beyond the Senior Centre and the shop, hundreds of older people also participate in the health-related activities of the Leisure Association, with rambling and swimming continuing to feature prominently in this programme.

Participation is not just about doing particular kinds of activities put on by a given organization – albeit in this instance activities largely established and run by older people themselves. Participation in the project has also been very much about participation as volunteers. Again, over the years, scores of older people have volunteered their services perhaps beginning very modestly by, for example, preparing food in the shop but then, as confidence and expertise has grown, moving onto other aspects such as being a CareLine volunteer or a peer health counsellor. Chapter 9 explored the experiences of some of these people, highlighting the various ways in which participation has been important to them, and how this changes and develops over time.

We would therefore contend that the project has been successful in meeting one of its original three aims of 'encouraging the involvement of more older people in health care programmes'. However, when we look closely at who it is who participates we might wish to question just how wide and inclusive that participation has been. For example, it was realized very early on in the project that older men were notable by their absence. Where they did participate, this

THE SELF HEALTH CARE
IN OLD AGE PROJECT

ACTION ELEMENT

RESEARCH ELEMENT

Aims:
1 To raise older people's awareness of
the need for health care and
maintenance.
2 To encourage the involvement of
more older people in health care
programmes.
3 To assist older people to identify
their health needs, and to develop
the skills and strategies they require
to obtain the resources to meet
their needs.

Aims:
1 To monitor the processes involved in
setting up the project, and in
developing its various elements over
the funding period.
2 To evaluate the impact of the project
on the self health care activities of
older people in North Staffordshire.

Activities:
1 A Peer Health Counselling scheme
2 A telephone link service (CareLine)
3 A variety of health-related courses
and activities
4 A Senior Health Shop

Foci:
1 The process of development
2 The collection of quantitive
information
3 The gathering of qualitative
information

SELF-EMPOWERED
HEALTH BEHAVIOUR

Internal criteria:
1 Participation
2 Accessibility
3 Informed choice
4 Skills development
5 Empowerment

European criteria:
1 Participation
2 Innovation
3 Cost-effectiveness

Figure 10.1   Action and research dimensions of the Self Health Care in Old Age
Project

was often as a result of being brought along by their wives – to the shop, to the
Look After Yourself course, and so on. Speculating on why this might be, we
concluded that it probably had to do with a combination of factors. These
include things like the 'image' which health promotion had at the time, with

many of the activities perceived as more suited to women than to men; the fact that the project being aimed at the over-fifties meant that, while many women had either retired or were not working, their husbands were often still in employment; and that the kinds of voluntary work on offer were much more about people skills as opposed to organizing, leading and managing – again, traditionally attracting more women than men.

Similarly, it has to be observed that participation by black and minority ethnic elders in the project was virtually non-existent. These concerns were discussed and debated regularly, and various efforts made to encourage and facilitate wider participation through links with community leaders of the Asian and West Indian communities in particular, and through putting on women-only and sometimes men-only sessions and activities and, for example, by having specific window displays in the shop of relevance to men's health concerns. As the project continued to develop, and later to spawn other associated activities such as advocacy work, much of what we had learnt was also applied to developing outreach activities (led by peer health counsellors in residential homes and sheltered housing complexes) rather than simply expecting that people would turn up and participate simply because the facilities existed. While such developments went some way towards addressing these dilemmas, the encouragement of participation by marginalized and excluded sectors of the older population still remains a crucial issue for the Foundation and for health promotion activities more generally. Inevitably too, these concerns about participation are intimately linked with accessibility.

How accessible has the project been?

In terms of *accessibility*, we endeavoured to ensure that accessing the various elements and activities in the project was as easy as possible for older people. Access is about knowledge and information; about physically being able to gain entry to an activity or place; and about a philosophy or way or working. With regard to information and knowledge, the description of the project in Chapter 5, together with some of the results of our monitoring and evaluation, show that great importance was placed on advertising what the project was doing through publicity material, through the local media, through a regular news-sheet and through a variety of dissemination activities. Word of mouth, while important, cannot be relied upon alone. The inherent dilemma here is in the balance to be struck between advertising and talking about what a project like this does, as opposed to getting on with the day-to-day running and development work. Again, this issue is one that the Foundation faced throughout the project, as well as in its activities both before and since.

Turning to physical access, it is important to record that the preparatory work that went in to siting the project was considerable. In the event, the location and indeed the size of the shop in particular were not ideal. Although the shop and the Senior Centre might be only five minutes away from the central bus station, they are five minutes away in opposite directions! So, ways had to be found to make links between the different elements in order for information to flow and for access to be facilitated. People may well walk in through the door if they know of a project or facility, but this is often very difficult to do if individuals lack confidence and do not know anybody. We have seen from some of the accounts in previous chapters how this has been addressed. Peer health counsellors, for example, have been on hand at both the centre and the shop in order to introduce newcomers to the facilities and activities. They have also accompanied people to the start of classes or courses where appropriate. In other words, the project developed a way of working which was about 'supported access'.

The shop itself was deliberately designed to be as inviting and welcoming as possible, and not to look like a clinic waiting room or, even, just an information centre. The provision of refreshments was a deliberate strategy to get people in through the door and this worked well for a considerable length of time. In addition, the shop was accessible in that, for many customers, it became a regular part of their daily or weekly activity schedule: when they were in Hanley to shop, they would call in.

Access was also facilitated through information provision. As we learnt in Chapter 9, access routes for the project's volunteers were many and varied: some learnt about what was on offer through the local press, others through existing voluntary work and contacts they had already made. However, once in the project, attempts were made to open up access to other volunteering opportunities according to the needs and demands of both the volunteers themselves, and of the evolving project.

Finally, we observed that access is crucially about a philosophy or way of working. Here, it is important to record that the project (and indeed the Foundation) has constantly striven to have as open an access policy and philosophy as possible. It has been a conscious decision, for example, to ensure that the centre, the shop and the Leisure Association do not have a fixed membership list (and by definition, no waiting lists).

What has informed choice meant?

Information is integrally related to both participation and to access. Older people, like all people, need information in order to be able to make choices in respect of their self health care activities as with other areas of their lives. The criteria of *informed choice* can therefore be seen to mean differing things in different contexts. Informed choice in the context of the shop has meant presenting information – both written and verbal – in appropriate ways. The racks of leaflets around the walls leave people free to choose whether or not to take them and, subsequently, to make an informed choice about whether there might be anything they wish to pursue further in terms of seeking more information, asking advice, joining an activity, putting themselves forward as a volunteer or whatever. Similarly, knowing that there are particular services on offer for which they do not have to make an appointment – blood pressure checking and weight monitoring for instance – leaves people free to choose whether or not to take up this opportunity.

Beyond making information available and accessible is the issue of whether or not people feel this facilitates them making informed choices. Again, our findings in Chapter 7 demonstrate some of the ways in which people say this has occurred, as they describe what they have done with the information in terms of their own diet, their activities or their dealings with professional health workers. These views also find further echoes in the reactions of participants to the things they have learnt on the Look After Yourself courses, and again in the discussion of volunteering in Chapter 9. Here, information giving through the training and ongoing support enables volunteers to make informed choices about what they would be most suited for and, as they develop, how they might best meet their own changing needs.

By means of information giving, ensuring access and encouraging participation, we would contend that the project has achieved its aim of 'raising older people's awareness of the need for health care and maintenance'. This, however, has been a largely bottom-up approach: listening, originally, to what older people said they needed and wanted and then creating the structures and activities through which it has been possible to deliver some of this information and thereby raise awareness. Awareness raising and the encouragement of involvement lead, inexorably, onto an examination of what, if any, skills people have been enabled to develop as a result of involvement with the project.

What skills have older people (and staff) developed?

Skills development in a project such as this is very difficult to assess and quantify. However, the qualitative evidence suggests that many of the older people who have had contact with the project have acquired identifiable practical skills as well as developing their confidence, self-esteem and sense of identity. In particular, they have developed the kinds of self health care skills outlined in Chapter 3, notably those relating to 'health information skills' and to 'disease prevention and health promotion skills' (Coppard *et al.* 1984). Visitors to the shop talk of the changes they have made to their lifestyles, and of the impact this has had on their dealings with health and social care professionals. Participants in the Look After Yourself courses and in many of the leisure activities talk similarly of the ways in which they have learnt to handle stress and tension, and the impact that exercise and activity has on their mood and well-being. Certainly then, we would contend that there is clear evidence from the research findings that older people have been enabled to develop a variety of skills.

Beyond this, however, it was argued in Chapter 3 that while self health care skills are important in individual terms, there is also a crucial element of developing and sharing these skills and knowledge with other people. We can point here to the development of interpersonal and communication skills, counselling skills and leadership skills. The experiences of the older volunteers involved in peer health counselling, CareLine and health-related activities at the Senior Centre and through the Leisure Association, as recorded in their own words in Chapter 9, are testimony to the ways in which they have grown in self-confidence as they enhance existing skills and learn new ones. The benefits of this in terms of their own health and well-being are manifest in the ways in which they talk about the satisfaction and enjoyment it brings, as well as 'having a purpose in life'. Again then, we would contend that the project has gone a considerable way towards achieving its third aim of 'assisting older people to identify their health needs, and to develop the skills and strategies they require to obtain the resources to meet their needs'.

Staff too have acquired, enhanced and developed skills. At the close of Chapter 9, we briefly discussed some of the ways in which this had happened. For me, it was very much an apprenticeship in the sense of learning how to translate my academic research skills into effective and appropriate ways of monitoring and evaluating a real live development project. For my more experienced developmental colleagues they became, by their own admission, much more research minded as a consequence of their close involvement in the choice, design and administration of the research tools, as well as in the ongoing analysis and application of the emerging findings. Today, the research literature tends to label this process with terms such as being 'critically reflective' or becoming a 'reflexive practitioner'. For us, we learnt as we went along that taking the time and giving ourselves permission to be reflective, was important to the overall development of the project, to our professional relationships with each other and with the older people with whom we worked. Our differing skills also contributed to us becoming more aware, as the project progressed, of the ways in which research and action can be complementary rather than each being pursued in the abstract.

Critically however, and with the benefit of hindsight, what becomes clear is that in many ways the project perpetuated some of the distinctions between 'us', the professionals, and 'them', the older people. Although striving to work *with* rather than for older people, there was still a clear demarcation in many instances in terms of professional boundaries and professional expertise and knowledge. This was particularly noticeable in terms of the research dimension in which, if the truth be told, it never really occurred to us to consider the possibility that the older people with whom we had contact might be not only participants and volunteers, but also fellow researchers. Indeed, one could argue that older people were still very much the 'objects' or 'subjects' of this action-research project.

How empowered have people become?

Finally in this summary, we come again to the thorny issue of *empowerment*. In Chapter 2, we discussed a variety of ways in which empowerment can be understood and operationalized, noting its close association with health promotion and community development work, and with education. We also observed that there are important distinctions to be made between individual, organizational and community level empowerment. At the individual level, it was suggested at the close of Chapter 3, that empowerment could be defined in terms of raising awareness, knowledge, understanding and competence, and that this conceptualization underlay the development of the Self Health Care in Old Age Project.

From the findings presented in Chapters 7, 8 and 9, it has become evident that while people who participated in the project do not use the term 'empowerment', they have indeed experienced many of the dimensions encapsulated by this term. Shop customers, for example, have had their awareness raised both through information and through discussions with staff. While the evaluation did not systematically assess people's changes in knowledge, understanding and competence through structured tests or questionnaires, there is qualitative evidence that people can identify ways in which their behaviour and actions have changed. Visitors to the shop talk about changes to their diet, and note how they have taken up exercise and other activities in attempts to improve both their physical and mental health and well-being. The unthreatening atmosphere, the food, the friendliness and the lack of time pressures have all facilitated this sense of empowerment.

Older participants in a variety of health-related activities, notably the Look After Yourself courses, also report changes which demonstrate individual empowerment. The stories recalled in Chapter 8 show how people have grown in self-confidence, how they have taken greater control of their own lives, learnt new things and expanded their horizons. They are also very articulate about the ways in which involvement has improved their health. These themes were also expanded upon by the older volunteers we met in Chapter 9. Rediscovering old skills and learning new things has enabled these individuals to become more aware of both their own, and others', health needs. They have found companionship through voluntary work, gained in self-confidence, enjoy what they do and find it fulfilling and challenging. Many of these changes echo the principles of empowerment outlined at the end of Chapter 2 (Barnes and Walker 1996).

However, one might still legitimately criticize the approach we took in this project for its overemphasis on individual level empowerment. The project's three main aims were indeed couched very much within an individual behaviour change model. Such individualization can, as was highlighted in Chapter 2, lead to the potential for victim blaming. This danger needs to be consciously avoided and addressed. While wider involvement at an organizational and community level was important to the project's overall development, effecting change at these levels was not a primary objective. The making of links between these levels is a key challenge for those working within this arena, and brings us back once again to the ways in which health promotion needs to be contextualized with wider social, environmental and political concerns.

Self Health Care in Old Age: lessons for practice

The evidence from our own work, together with the case studies presented in Chapter 4, suggests that projects and programmes aimed at enhancing the health and well-being of older people share some common features and, by implication, important lessons for practice. In the mid-1980s, David Macfadyen, the then manager for the World Health Organization's Global Programme on Health of the Elderly, observed that self health programmes had four features in common: their setting, the ways in which they were publicized, the involvement of older people and multiple sponsorship (Macfadyen 1985). From our own experience, we would add four further issues which we regard as important for the practice of these kinds of health promotion with older people: the need to consider professional inputs, training and resources, research and evaluation, and time. These eight sets of 'lessons for practice' are briefly considered in turn below.

Setting

It is evident that the exhortation to 'begin where people are' in the development of health promotion activities with older people is one that can be taken both literally and metaphorically. Literally, many of the self health care programmes and projects discussed build on settings which are familiar and comfortable to older people. They are often community centred and often have a very strong social, as opposed to strictly health-oriented, flavour. They illustrate the importance of social activity in the lives of older people, the great diversity in suitable settings, and the ways in which health is indivisible from many other aspects of people's everyday lives. In practice terms, this means that at the very least we should be alert to the great variety of contexts within which health promotion with older people might take place.

Publicity

Many programmes and projects have been reliant, initially at least, on vigorous publicity at a very local level. Reaching out to people who are often not considered as legitimate targets of health promotion means responding in ways that will engage their interest and encourage them to become and stay involved. The examples discussed in this book have made use of the whole gamut of publicity techniques available these days, from conventional leafleting campaigns through to interactive video and television programming. They also illustrate how important it is to continue to invest in publicity if a project is to go on developing and attracting new people and new ideas, rather than becoming moribund. In essence, the key lesson here concerns the means and resources needed to sustain such health promotion programmes.

Involvement of older people

The recurrent phrase in all these programmes and projects is that they have worked *with*, not just *for* older people. They all began through a combination of bright ideas and self-defined needs, rather than by imposing a top-down, professionally led model of health promotion and education. The projects reveal the ways in which older people are involved in so many facets of programme development: in planning, in implementation, as volunteers or peer educators, as participants, as instructors and group facilitators, as advisers, as publicists, and as co-workers and co-researchers. They also demonstrate that it is possible to attract and involve non-traditional groups of older people in self health care activities and in finding their own solutions to their own problems. Self health initiatives are not, and need not be, solely white middle-class activities.

   The lessons for health promotion practice are clear in terms of the requirement to seek out health needs as defined by older people themselves, and to actively involve people in formulating the most appropriate ways of addressing those needs. If successful this should lead, in turn, to the development of a culture of participation in which people choose to remain involved because they themselves identify what benefits they gain. This is manifestly different from didactic approaches to health promotion in which people are told or instructed what to do in order to improve their health, and are then expected to go away and do it. This also chimes with the broader points made in Chapter 2 about the dangers of many health promotion activities being too prescriptive.

Multiple sponsorship

The programmes and projects discussed in these pages are patently not the preserve of one funding agency or sponsoring body. Indeed, multiple sponsorship is what characterizes these initiatives, and sponsorship which involves not purely financial support but sponsorship-in-kind. This may involve the provision of things like transport for people to attend health courses, the arranging of appropriate venues, or offering to publicize what is on offer. Collaboration between government agencies (at local and national levels), public and voluntary organizations and lay groups appears to be commonplace in these developments. This multifaceted approach suggests that we have much to learn from the ways in which self health care projects have enabled barriers between statutory and voluntary agencies, and between private and public concerns, to be effectively bridged. In these contexts, self health care has not been the preserve of any one service or sponsor but, instead, has drawn on and utilized a range of expertise and experience.

More negatively, many projects and programmes suffer from financial support being too time limited. The evidence is that health promotion interventions take considerable time to yield substantive benefits and outcomes. While some initiatives may be able to move towards a position of being totally or partially self-sufficient after a number of years, others falter. This concern is also a strategic one and is returned to again when we consider the issue of time more generally below.

Professional inputs

As with sponsorship, it is evident that the programmes and projects reviewed here have all involved collaboration between professionals and lay people. Key professionals, often with community development skills in addition to their main health-related area of interest, have featured in all these initiatives. Professionals, academics, students and older people work together to ensure that the projects become well established in their local communities. Three lessons for practice in particular stand out here: first, there is a need for much greater investment in training and education for staff who work with older people, and this should, logically, begin with an examination of the attitudes and motivations people have for this kind of work. Second, as projects continue to grow and develop, there is evidence that they need to rely less and less on professional inputs. As was pointed out in Chapter 2, excessive professionalization would therefore be counter-productive, although continuing professional inputs at some level also seem to be necessary. Third, this is essentially about a facilitative way of working with older people, and really needs to become a legitimate and recognized part of the job of the professional as opposed to being something done in, around and on top of everything else.

Training and resources

The shift noted above to working with instead of for people leads to a concomitant reorientation of the ways in which training is both conceived and delivered. The top-down, didactic approach of much health promotion has given way to a collaborative, bottom-up model with much more emphasis on group processes and active participation. We have seen, for example, that older volunteers do not tend to be recruited through the more familiar channels of work or family contacts. Rather, we found the local press and media to be very important, although word-of-mouth will probably always remain the most effective method. Once recruited, we come to the issue of training and support. It is often suggested that recruitment and training of older people is not worthwhile, that they require more training, and that it is not cost effective. On the contrary, our experience and that of others suggest that older volunteers repay the training and support they receive by putting in more time than other groups and by staying longer. Offering training and ongoing support is also one way in which volunteers are acknowledged and recognized, and their contributions valued. Alongside this has come the recognition that good quality aids, resources and access to materials are as important for older people as young people. Harnessing and enhancing the skills and abilities of those with the accumulated experience of many years of acting as natural helpers or as leaders of various kinds, shows how it is possible to maximize the potential of older people as health resources for their peers.

Research and evaluation

Although still at a relatively modest level, these projects reveal the importance of engaging in monitoring and evaluation, both in terms of continuing project development and as a way of disseminating findings to wider and more diverse audiences. The examples given here illustrate just how complex and sensitive research in these situations is. It needs to be integrated with the development of the project, to be both formative in the sense of providing regular feedback, as well as summative. We saw, for example, how the Foundation attempted to adapt and apply research methods and tools to fit the needs of particular elements in the project, as opposed to sticking rigidly to a classical model of evaluation. Non-intrusive and non-threatening techniques are required to research and evaluate developments such as these: techniques which will yield a combination of quantitative and qualitative data, and which convey the dynamic process of project development in addition to the health promotion outcomes (Nutbeam 1998).

Moreover, whatever the emphasis of the research, it is patently clear that certain steps have to be taken to set up and then carry out an action research project. Adequate preparation and groundwork are essential, with research strategies needing to be written in alongside the development proposals. This is often a condition of external funding as indeed it was in the Self Health Care in Old Age Project. Aims and objectives too have to be intelligible, explicit and above all realistic in terms of what can be achieved within a given time frame, and within the available resources of both people and finance.

Dissemination strategies too, both internal and external, have to be built in from the beginning, in order to keep people informed about what is going on, to ensure that needed changes are acted upon and that, externally, others can learn from, and possibly replicate, what has been done. Finally research, like development, is not a value-free undertaking. An action research project like the Self Health Care in Old Age one is something to which the whole organization has to have a commitment.

This presents a considerable challenge to conventional social scientific and epidemiological research methodology, and is an area ripe for much further development. Recent work is showing that with appropriate training and support, older people are just as capable as professionals of developing the requisite skills to carry out the kind of research described in this book (see, for example, Cooper *et al.* 1994; Tozer and Thornton 1995; Barnes 1999). Extending the roles of older people to include them as co-researchers in self health care projects may, in itself, contribute to their improved health and well-being. As yet, however, this remains purely at a speculative level.

Time

Perhaps the overriding feature common to all these projects is the considerable time and indeed patience which are needed for their development. The notion of being able to take down a pre-packaged programme of health education or promotion off-the-shelf, introduce it to a group of older people, and let it take its inevitable and successful course is completely unrealistic. Detailed and adequate work on the ground, in the communities where older people live, is vital to gain an understanding and appreciation of the ways in which health underscores their lives. Gaining access, listening, working alongside, supporting and cajoling are skilled and time-consuming activities but vitally necessary if we are to make a reality of the notions of empowerment and participation. They are also critical to the longer-term aims of many of these projects, which are striving to become self-sustaining beyond the formal input of professionals and of initial funds.

Self Health Care in Old Age: lessons for policy

Distilling lessons for policy from the developments outlined in this book is patently a difficult task. It is also, of necessity, likely to be highly selective. However, with the transition to a new millennium, with the mid-term Labour government currently championing older people's issues (through its Inter-Ministerial Group on Ageing and initiatives such as Better Government for Older People) and with the UK population containing more older people than ever before, there is a momentum which cannot be ignored. Thus, in moving towards the close of this book, we attempt to flag up three areas which, from the evidence discussed in these pages, lead to the view that the time has never been more appropriate to move older people and health promotion issues centre-stage in contemporary policy debates. The three areas focused on are the need to reinstate community development approaches as key to health promotion policy for older people; the need for older people to be fully recognized as a central resource in health promotion not only for themselves and their peers, but also for society at large; and the need for health policy to be preventive and holistic as opposed to curative.

Self health care as community development

Unfashionable though it may be, one of the main messages of this book is that a community development approach to health promotion works well with older people. This approach requires professionals to work closely with communities – in this case communities of older people – in order to identify particular problems and resources in respect of older people's health; to work out appropriate responses and interventions; to articulate how success can be gauged; and to learn and disseminate the wider lessons. Such approaches fell out of favour in the UK during the Thatcher years (1979–90), partly because they clearly did not mesh with the economically driven agendas in health, and partly because they were associated with a political radicalism which was almost diametrically opposed to the policies and practices of the New Right (Killoran *et al.* 1997). A further criticism noted at the beginning of our consideration of self health care (see Chapter 3) was that such developments were poorly evaluated if at all. Today, the climate for reappraising and reinstating these kinds of approaches seems more promising for a number of reasons.

First, health issues and health policy are more clearly entwined with social and environmental factors, and with social policy than ever before. Especially where older people are concerned, it is increasingly unhelpful to perpetuate these distinctions and to demarcate rigid boundaries between health and social needs. The accumulation of the kinds of research reviewed in earlier chapters shows, for example, just how important social support and social networks are to older people's health and well-being, and how family, friends and the wider community all contribute (Phillipson *et al.* 1998). Policy which supports a community development approach to health promotion can surely only enhance and develop the 'health protecting' effects of these networks of support, mutual help and friendship. The Foundation's project and others are thus designed not to replace or displace formal services, but to complement them.

The second reason for believing that community development approaches have much to offer concerns the current emphasis in all public policy on consultation, consumerism and empowerment. Towards the end of 1998, the government's Inter-Ministerial Group produced a publication entitled *Building a Better Britain for Older People* (Department of Social Security (DSS) 1998). In his foreword, Prime Minister Tony Blair noted that the contributions of older people have 'not always been properly recognised by society or governments' and that one of the consequences of this is that 'their voices are ignored'. He went on to say that 'we must take the wishes and needs of older people seriously'; improving consultation was identified as a key strategy for achieving this. This governmental view now chimes very closely with the kinds of values that have underpinned much of the work on self health care. Indeed, many of the informants to the Health Education Authority's policy review on promoting the health of older people regarded direct consultation with older people as indispensable (Killoran *et al.* 1997). Moreover, a willingness to link policy development with an overt value base and 'culture of empowerment' (Walker 1998) is, as highlighted elsewhere, of crucial importance to future policy making (Bernard and Phillips 1998).

Third, and following on from the above, there now seems to be a greater recognition of the potential for research to inform policy. Although community development approaches may have fallen out of favour, they never actually disappeared as a method of working with people in local communities. Over the years, the research which has been done – piecemeal though it still may be – has shown how effective community development approaches are for hearing the voices of older people, for encouraging community-based participation and for facilitating people to comment critically on existing policies and provisions (Croft and Beresford 1990; Cooper *et al.* 1994; Church 1995; Tozer and Thornton 1995; Walker and Warren 1996; Barnes and Warren 1999). Given that public health concerns and health promotion are firmly back on the policy agenda, then this has, logically, to include the perspectives and needs of older people. Learning, and applying the lessons from their experiences, will help develop the two-way flow of information that is required if new policy initiatives promoting the health of older people are to have any lasting effect.

These three sets of reasons suggest that it is high time that older people's needs are now placed centre stage, not simply so they can be further singled out and pathologized as a problematic group, but so that they can legitimately be regarded as fully participating citizens, and considered as a resource for society at large. This is the second lesson for policy we consider below.

Older people as a resource

It will probably not have escaped readers' notice that volunteering – and volunteering by older people in particular – is at the heart of the present government's attempt to raise the profile of older people as fully participating citizens. 'Active ageing', as it is now being termed, is one of the priorities for the Inter-Ministerial Group (along with health and care issues, and participation and consultation). Moreover, the most recent national volunteering initiative was launched in the late spring of 1999. Behind the rhetoric though, what can the development and encouragement of such a policy of 'active ageing' learn from the findings about volunteering in the kinds of health promotion projects reported in this book?

First, in order for old age to be seen as a time of opportunity, various barriers to older people's involvement in volunteering and, indeed, in health promoting and leisure activities more generally, need to be overcome. These barriers include things like levels of previous education, people's financial circumstances, their reduced mobility and their health status. In addition, older people's uptake of opportunities will also be affected by the attitudes of the people whom they might encounter in such environments, and by organizational barriers to involvement. The Carnegie study, for example (Davis Smith 1992), revealed that one-fifth of organizations had a retirement age for volunteers, and 10 per cent experienced difficulties with insuring older volunteers, particularly for driving. Age discrimination, then, is something which clearly needs to be addressed by policy makers if opportunities for volunteering and for the involvement of more older people in health promotion activities are to be enhanced.

Second, once people do volunteer, our experience with the Self Health Care in Old Age Project shows that individuals want to be able to find a niche within which they are comfortable – to do the kind of voluntary work which they find personally satisfying, rather than being channelled into dead-end activities that nobody else wishes to do. Linked with this, it is also important to recognize that older people have skills and abilities which, in many instances, are going to waste. Like other groups, they want activities which will fulfil and develop them as people (while accepting too that, on occasion, volunteering is also likely to be boring and routine). For some, this may mean voluntary activities which most equate with their working lives, perhaps providing a structured environment, time commitments on a regular basis and so on. For many others though, this would be a disincentive, and organizations trying to attract older volunteers on the basis that it provides a continuation of paid work (albeit without financial remuneration) may in fact be mistaken. Moreover, the research we have done over the years reveals just how important 'challenge' is to volunteers' sense of self-fulfilment and satisfaction with what they do. Far too often, however, what we offer to older people is geared to their incompetencies and limitations, rather than building on their skills and experiences.

Third, offering support and training is one avenue through which it is possible to convey the value we place on older volunteers; ensuring that the environment is conducive to the work, and that people are recognized on a daily basis for what they are offering, are also vital. This touches on the vexed question of financial resources, and whether or not volunteers should be paid. The Foundation has always subscribed to the view that part of valuing the contribution of volunteers means covering out-of-pocket expenses (including travel, meals and things like telephone calls), although it does not actually pay people for their time. Nor, like some organizations, does it require volunteers to pay their own training expenses.

A policy of 'active ageing', in which volunteering is central to wider health promoting activities, needs to address a whole package through from the recruitment of older people to training and ongoing support. It also needs to be integrated with the points made above about health promotion policy and older people. If, for example, making older people's health is a priority for the New Health Action Zones (DSS 1998) where will voluntary action by older people feature? From our experience, it would seem that older people would be especially well placed to make a major contribution to the proposed Healthy Living Centres in each zone, undertaking precisely the kinds of roles, responsibilities and activities we have already documented here.

Preventive and holistic health policy

The third area to focus on is the need for health policy to be oriented around a comprehensive holistic and preventive focus. The opening chapters of this book traced the policy developments of the past one hundred years or so, noting the way in which public health concerns have re-emerged at the end of the twentieth century. The kinds of preventive, health promoting activities outlined in successive chapters throw into sharp relief yet again the close interconnections between individual health and well-being and the widening inequalities in society which impact negatively on people's health (Acheson 1998). These societal causes of ill health include things such as poverty, poor living conditions, unemployment and pollution. It was also noted how older people in particular are ill served and disadvantaged by many of the ways in which 'health' is currently delivered to the populace: they suffer from both overt and covert age discrimination; are negatively stereotyped as dependent, sick and ill; and felt to be beyond the reach, and not in need of, much health promotion activity. The key here is, as was pointed out at the start, to tread that fine line between challenging such views while at the same time not falling into the trap of replacing one set of stereotypes and images with more positive, but potentially equally damaging ones.

The kinds of health promoting activities undertaken by the older people discussed in this book are undoubtedly important for helping us to counter the negative imagery associated with growing older. However, it is still unfortunately the case that much of what has been outlined remains couched in an individual behaviour change model. While this should not be belittled in terms of the obvious changes it has made to the lives of the people we have encountered, wider improvements in terms of public health will come about only if the connections are made at a policy level between these kinds of individual activities, and the need to change aspects of the wider environment in which we all live and which we know to be harmful to health. Moreover, such policies must not pitch preventive and health promoting approaches in opposition to curative medicine but would, rather, both be part of a whole health strategy (Ashton and Seymour 1993). This is not to deny or minimize the potential conflicts of interest that might arise, but to highlight yet again that where older people are concerned, there is much to be said for a refocusing of resources into preventive activity (Bernard *et al.* 1993). A comprehensive preventive public health policy, delivered at a community level and linked with a strategy which emphasizes the promotion and maintenance of abilities in old age, as well as (but not instead of) targets for reducing the incidence of ill health and disability, is now long overdue.

Conclusion: an integrated policy approach

Finally, all that has been said above leads inexorably to the conclusion that developing health promotion policy for older people has to be but one element of an integrated, intersectoral policy approach. It is patently clear that the maintenance of health and well-being in old age is contingent upon a whole host of other factors: health and functional status, lifestyle, environment, service use, mobility, personality and motivation, social support, and attitudes, to name but a few. As was suggested in Chapter 2, this means that policy changes in arenas other than health are likely to have considerable, and perhaps unintended impacts. This also means that the interconnections have to be made very explicit. The consultative paper *Building a Better Britain for Older People* (DSS 1998) headlines a series of key areas which need to be addressed. Beginning with healthy living, it goes on to consider income, employment, travel, living environments, crime, care, and active lives, while Tony Blair's foreword claims that he will 'make sure the Government as a whole works together to respond to them'. Translating this rhetoric into practice will require intersectoral and inter-agency working, within a multi-perspective framework (Killoran *et al.* 1997) which makes older people's self-care and health promotion needs, as well as the resources they bring, a central consideration. Achieving this will not be easy, but if health promotion, public health and healthy living ideals are to be an important element of the new policy agenda in the twenty-first century, then it is high time that older people were party to these developments at both local and national levels.

References

Acheson, D. (1998) *Inequalities in Health*. London: HMSO.
Action for Health (1988) *Initiation in Local Communities*. London: Community Projects Foundation.
Adams, R. (1990) *Self Help, Social Work and Empowerment*. London: Macmillan.
Ahmad, W.I.U., Kernohan, E.E.M. and Baker, M.R. (1989) Health of British Asians: a research review, *Community Medicine*, 11(1): 49–56.
Anderson, J. (1986) Health skills: the power to choose, *Health Education Journal*, 45(1): 19–24.
Andrews, G. (1990) Role of primary health care for the elderly, in R.L. Kane, J. Grimley Evans and D. Macfadyen (eds) *Improving the Health of Older People: A World View*. Oxford: Oxford University Press.
Animation and Dissemination Service (1985) The European Programme to Combat Poverty (Elderly People). Unpublished information pack. London: Age Concern England.
Antonovsky, A. (1984) The sense of coherence as a determinant of health, in J.P. Matarazzo (ed.) *Behavioural Health*. New York: Wiley.
Antonovsky, A. (1987) *Unravelling the Mystery of Health: How People Manage Others and Stay Well*. New York: Wiley.
Antonovsky, A. (1996) The salutogenic model as a theory to guide health promotion, *Health Promotion International*, 11(1): 11–18.
Arber, S. and Ginn, J. (1991) *Gender and Later Life: A Sociological Analysis of Resources and Constraints*. London: Sage.
Arendt, H. (1958) *The Human Condition*. Chicago: University of Chicago Press.
Ashton, J. and Seymour, H. (1988) *The New Public Health*. Milton Keynes: Open University Press.
Ashton, J. and Seymour, H. (1993) The setting for a new public health, in A. Beattie, M. Gott, L. Jones and M. Sidell (eds) *Health and Wellbeing: A Reader*. London: Macmillan.
Ashton, L. (1995) 'Ageing Well': a new health programme in the UK, *Elders – The Journal of Care and Practice*, 4(2): 17–30.
Atkin, K. (1998) Ageing in a multi-racial Britain: demography, policy and practice, in

M. Bernard and J. Phillips (eds) *The Social Policy of Old Age: Moving into the 21st Century*. London: Centre for Policy on Ageing.

Backett, K. and Davison, C. (1992) Rationale or reasonable? Perceptions of health at different stages of life, *Health Education Journal*, 51(2).

Balarajan, R. (1995) Ethnicity and variations in the nation's health, *Health Trends*, 27: 114–19.

Balarajan, R. and Raleigh, V. (1997) Patterns of mortality among Bangladeshis in England and Wales, *Ethnicity and Health*, 2: 1–2.

Ball, M. (1988) *Evaluation in the Voluntary Sector*. London: Forbes Trust.

Ball, M. and Bernard, M. (1987) Monitoring as a way to improve our practice, in M. Bernard (ed.) *Developing Services for Elderly Mentally Infirm People: Responses to the 'Rising Tide' Initiative*. Stoke-on-Trent: Beth Johnson Foundation in association with Adult and Continuing Education Department, Keele University.

Banister, P., Burman, E., Parker, I., Taylor, M. and Tindall, C. (1994) *Qualitative Methods in Psychology: A Research Guide*. Buckingham: Open University Press.

Barnes, M. (1999) Working with older people to evaluate the Fife User Panels Project, in M. Barnes and L. Warren (eds) *Paths to Empowerment*. Bristol: Policy Press.

Barnes, M. and Walker, A. (1996) Consumerism versus empowerment: a principled approach to the involvement of older service users, *Policy and Politics*, 24(4): 375–93.

Barnes, M. and Warren, L. (eds) (1999) *Paths to Empowerment*. Bristol: Policy Press.

Beattie, A. (1984) Health education and the science teacher: invitation to a debate, *Education and Health*, 2(1): 9–15.

Beattie, A. (1991) The evaluation of community development initiatives in health promotion: a review of current strategies, in *'Roots and Branches': Papers from the OU/HEA 1990 Winter School on Community Development and Health*. Milton Keynes: Health Education Unit/The Open University.

Beattie, A. (1997a) *The Views of Housebound Older People*, Briefing paper no. 1. London: Age Concern England.

Beattie, A. (1997b) *The Views of Black and Minority Ethnic Older People*, Briefing paper no. 3. London: Age Concern England.

Beattie, A., Jones, L. and Sidell, M. (1992) *Health and Wellbeing*. K258, second level distance learning course. Milton Keynes: The Open University.

Bebbington, A.C. (1988) The expectation of life without disability in England and Wales, *Social Science and Medicine*, 27(4): 321–7.

Beeker, C., Guenther-Grey, C. and Raj, A. (1998) Community empowerment paradigm drift and the primary prevention of HIV/AIDS, *Social Science and Medicine*, 46(7): 831–42.

Bennett, G.J. and Ebrahim, S. (1995) *The Essentials of Health Care in Old Age*, 2nd edn. London: Edward Arnold.

Benzeval, M., Judge, K. and Whitehead, M. (1995) *Tackling Inequalities in Health: An Agenda for Action*. London: King's Fund.

Beresford, P. and Croft, S. (1993) *Citizen Involvement: A Practical Guide for Change*. London: Macmillan.

Bernard, M. (1983) Easing the burden, *Community Care*, 27 October: 23–5.

Bernard, M. (1984a) Voluntary care for the elderly mentally infirm and their relatives: a British example, *The Gerontologist*, 24(2): 116–19.

Bernard, M. (ed.) (1984b) *Leisure in Later Life: Examples of Community Based Initiatives*. Stoke-on-Trent: Beth Johnson Foundation.

Bernard, M. (1988) Taking charge: strategies for self-empowered health behaviour among older people, *Health Education Journal*, 47(2/3): 87–90.

Bernard, M. (1989) Research in action: self health care and older people, *Hygie – International Journal of Health Education*, 8(2): 11–15.

Bernard, M. (1992) *Evaluating Voluntary Action*. Stoke-on-Trent: Evaluation Research Unit, Keele University.

Bernard, M. (1993) Findings of a UK project on older volunteers – *Healthy Ageing: A UK Model Programme*. Round table, World Congress of Gerontology, Budapest, Hungary, 4–9 July.

Bernard, M. (1998) The Beth Johnson Foundation: a quarter of a century of research with, for and about older people, *Education and Ageing*, 13(2): 143–62.

Bernard, M. and Ivers, V. (1986) Peer health counselling: a way of countering dependency?, in C. Phillipson, M. Bernard and P. Strang (eds) *Dependency and Inter-dependency in Old Age: Theoretical Perspectives and Policy Alternatives*. London: Croom Helm.

Bernard, M. and Meade, K. (1993) Perspectives on the lives of older women, in M. Bernard and K. Meade (eds) *Women Come of Age: Perspectives on the Lives of Older Women*. London: Edward Arnold.

Bernard, M. and Phillips, J. (1998) Ageing in tomorrow's Britain, in M. Bernard and J. Phillips (eds) *The Social Policy of Old Age: Moving into the 21st Century*. London: Centre for Policy on Ageing.

Bernard, M. and Phillipson, C. (1991) Self-care and health in old age, in S.J. Redfern (ed.) *Nursing Elderly People*, 2nd edn. Edinburgh: Churchill Livingstone.

Bernard, M., Smith, J. and Tomkinson, S. (1983) *The Potteries Elderly Support Group: An Example of Voluntary Care for the Elderly Mentally Infirm and their Relatives*. Stoke-on-Trent: Beth Johnson Foundation.

Bernard, M., Meade, K. and Tinker, A. (1993) Women come of age, in M. Bernard and K. Meade (eds) *Women Come of Age: Perspectives on the Lives of Older Women*. London: Edward Arnold.

Bernard, M., Johnson, N. and Waterson, J. (1994) Monitoring and evaluation: a key issue for voluntary groups, *Social Services Research*, 4(Nov./Dec.): 47–59.

Biggs, S., Bernard, M., Kingston, P. and Nettleton, H. (1998) *The Health Impact of Age-Specific Housing*, interim report to West Midlands Regional Health Authority. Stoke-on-Trent: Keele University.

Birmingham Voluntary Services Council (1989) *Evaluation for Voluntary Organisations*. Birmingham: Birmingham Voluntary Services Council.

Blakemore, K. (1998) *Social Policy: An Introduction*. Buckingham: Open University Press.

Blakemore, K. and Boneham, M. (1993) *Age, Race and Ethnicity: A Comparative Approach*. Buckingham: Open University Press.

Blane, D., Brunner, E. and Wilkinson, R. (eds) (1996) *Health and Social Organization: Towards a Health Policy for the 21st Century*. London: Routledge.

Blaxter, M. (1983) The causes of disease: women talking, *Social Science and Medicine*, 17: 59–69.

Blaxter, M. (1990) *Health and Lifestyles*. London: Tavistock/Routledge.

Blaxter, M. (1996) The significance of socioeconomic factors in health for medical care and the National Health Service, in D. Blane, E. Brunner and R. Wilkinson (eds) *Health and Social Organization: Towards a Health Policy for the 21st Century*. London: Routledge.

Blaxter, M. and Paterson, L. (1982) *Mothers and Daughters: A Three-Generational Study of Health, Attitudes and Behaviour*. Oxford: Heinemann Educational.

Bodie, L. (1997) *The Views of Older People Expressed through Focus Groups*, Briefing paper no. 2. London: Age Concern England.

Bond, J. and Coleman, P. (1993) Ageing into the twenty-first century, in J. Bond, P. Coleman and S. Peace (eds) *Ageing in Society – An Introduction to Social Gerontology*, 2nd edn. London: Sage.

Bone, M., Bebbington, A., Jagger, C., Morgan, K. and Nicolaas, G. (1995) *Health Expectancy and its Uses*. London: HMSO.

Brannen, J. (ed.) (1992) *Mixing Methods: Qualitative and Quantitative Research*. Aldershot: Avebury.

Braye, S. and Preston-Shoot, M. (1995) *Empowering Practice in Social Care*. Buckingham: Open University Press.

British Geriatrics Society (1993) Health promotion in later life. Statement from the British Geriatrics Society for the Health of the Aged. London: Royal College of Physicians.

Broad, B. and Fletcher, C. (eds) (1993) *Practitioner Social Work Research in Action*. London: Whiting and Birch.

Browne, C.V. (1995) Empowerment in social work practice with older women, *Social Work*, 40(3): 358–64.

Browne, C.V. (1998) *Women, Feminism and Aging*. New York: Springer.

Bryman, A. (1988) *Quantity and Quality in Social Research*. London: Unwin Hyman.

Bryman, A. (1992) Quantitative and qualitative research: further reflections on their integration, in J. Brannen (ed.) *Mixing Methods: Qualitative and Quantitative Research*. Aldershot: Avebury.

Bunton, R. (1993) Health promotion as social policy, in R. Bunton and G. Macdonald (eds) *Health Promotion: Disciplines and Diversity*. London: Routledge.

Bury, M. (1988) Arguments about ageing: long life and its consequences, in N. Wells and C. Freer (eds) *The Ageing Population: Burden or Challenge?* London: Macmillan.

Butler, R.N. and Gleason, H. (eds) (1985) *Productive Aging: Enhancing Vitality in Later Life*. New York: Springer.

Butler, R.N., Gertman, J.S., Oberlander, D.L. and Schindler, L. (1979) Self-care, self-help, and the elderly, *International Journal of Aging and Human Development*, 10(1): 95–119.

Bytheway, B. (1982) Fries and Crapo review symposium: ageing and the rectangular survival curve, *Ageing and Society*, 2(2): 389–91.

Calnan, M. (1987) *Health and Illness*. London: Tavistock.

Carr, W. and Kemmis, S. (1986) *Becoming Critical: Education, Knowledge and Action Research*. London: Falmer Press.

Chambre, S.M. (1987) *Good Deeds in Old Age: Volunteering by the New Leisure Class*. Lexington, MA: Lexington Books.

Chambre, S.M. (1993) Volunteerism by elders: past trends and future prospects, *The Gerontologist*, 33(2): 221–8.

Charlton, J., Wallace, M. and White, I. (1994) Long term illness: results from the 1991 census, *Population Trends*, 75: 19–25.

Cheetham, J., Fuller, R., McIvor, G. and Petch, A. (1992) *Evaluating Social Work Effectiveness*. Buckingham: Open University Press.

Church, K. (1995) *Forbidden Narratives: Critical Autobiography as Science*. Toronto: Gordon Breach.

Cockerham, W.C., Sharp, K. and Wilcox, J.A. (1983) Ageing and perceived health status, *Journal of Gerontology*, 38(3): 349–55.

Coleman, A. and Chira, T. (1991) *Coping with Change: Focus on Retirement*. London: Health Education Authority.

Cooper, M., Sidell, M. and Lewisham Older Women's Health Survey Project (1994) *Lewisham Older Women's Health Survey*. London: EdROP The City Lit.

Cooperstock, R. (1979) Sex differences in psychotropic drug use, *Social Science and Medicine*, 12b: 179–86.

Coppard, L.C., White-Riley, M., Macfadyen, D.M. and Dean, K. (1984) *Self Health Care and Older People: A Manual for Public Policy and Programme Development*. Copenhagen: World Health Organisation.

Corbin, J. and Strauss, A. (1988) *Unending Work and Care: Managing Chronic Illness at Home*. San Francisco, CA: Jossey-Bass.

Corey, S. (1953) *Action Research to Improve School Practice*. New York: Teachers College, Columbia University.

Cornwell, J. (1984) *Hard Earned Lives: Accounts of Health and Illness from East London*. London: Tavistock.

Cox, B.D., Blaxter, M., Buckle, A.L.J., *et al.* (1987) *The Health and Lifestyle Survey*. London: Health Promotion Research Trust.

Cox, E.O. and Parsons, R.J. (1994) *Empowerment-Oriented Social Work Practice with the Elderly*. Pacific Grove, CA: Brooks/Cole.

Craig, G. and Mayo, M. (eds) (1995) *Community Empowerment: A Reader in Participation and Development*. London: Zed Books.

Creber, A., Ivers, V. and Bernard, M. (1985) Self-health care in old age: a proposal. Unpublished paper. Stoke-on-Trent: Beth Johnson Foundation.

Crimmins, E.M., Saito,Y. and Ingegneri, D. (1989) Changes in life expectancy and disability-free life expectancy in the United States, *Population and Development Review*, 15(2): 235–67.

Croft, S. and Beresford, P. (1990) *From Paternalism to Participation: Involving People in Social Services*. London: Open Services Project and Joseph Rowntree Foundation.

Croft, S. and Beresford, P. (1992) The politics of participation, *Critical Social Policy*, 2(2): 20–44.

Croft, S. and Beresford, P. (1995) Whose empowerment? Equalising the competing discourses in community care, in R. Jack (ed.) *Empowerment in Community Care*. London: Chapman and Hall.

Cusack, S. (1998) Leadership in seniors' centres: power and empowerment in relations between seniors and staff, *Education and Ageing*, 13(1): 49–66.

Cusack, S. and Thompson, W. (1995) *Mental Fitness: A Critical Component of Healthy Aging*, summary report of a Community Research and Development Project, in consultation with the Lifelong Learning Advisory Group Century House. New Westminster, BC: Parks and Recreation.

Cusack, S. and Thompson, W. (1996) *The Mental Fitness Pilot Project: A Summary Report*, Lifelong Learning Committee. New Westminster, BC: Century House.

Dalley, G. (1998) Health and social welfare policy, in M. Bernard and J. Phillips (eds) *The Social Policy of Old Age: Moving Into the 21st Century*. London: Centre for Policy on Ageing.

Dalley, G., Howse, K., Killoran, A. and Seal, H. (1996) *A Framework for Promoting the Health of Older People: A Discussion Document*. London: Health Education Authority and Centre for Policy on Ageing.

Davis Smith, J. (1992) *Volunteering: Widening Horizons in the Third Age*, research paper no. 7, Carnegie Inquiry into the Third Age. Dunfermline: Carnegie UK Trust.

Davis Smith, J. (1998) *The 1997 National Survey of Volunteering*. London: National Centre for Volunteering.

Davison, C. and Davey Smith, G. (1995) The baby and the bath water: examining socio-cultural and free-market critiques of health promotion, in R. Bunton, S. Nettleton and R. Burrows (eds) *The Sociology of Health Promotion: Critical Analyses of Consumption, Lifestyle and Risk*. London: Routledge.

Deakin, J. (1998) Older people as volunteers: burden of dependency or carers in the community? Unpublished undergraduate dissertation, Department of Applied Social Studies, Keele University.

Dean, K. (1983) Self-care: what people do for themselves, in S. Hatch and I. Kickbusch (eds) *Self-Help and Health in Europe: New Approaches in Health Care*. Copenhagen: World Health Organisation.

Dean, K. (1986) Self-care behaviour: implications for aging, in K. Dean, T. Hickey and B.E. Holstein (eds) *Self-Care and Health in Old Age: Health Behaviour Implications for Policy and Practice*. London: Croom Helm.

Dean, K. (1989) Conceptual, theoretical and methodological issues in self-care research, *Social Science and Medicine*, 29(2): 117–23.

Dean, K. (1992) Health-related behaviour: concepts and methods, in M.G. Ory, R.P. Abeles and P.D. Lipman (eds) *Aging, Health and Behaviour*. London: Sage.

Dean, K., Hickey, T. and Holstein, B.E. (eds) (1986) *Self-Care and Health in Old Age: Health Behaviour Implications for Policy and Practice*. London: Croom Helm.

Denzin, N.K. and Lincoln, Y.S. (eds) (1994) *Handbook of Qualitative Research*. London: Sage.

Department of Health (DoH) (1991) *The Patients' Charter*. London: DoH.

Department of Health (DoH) (1992) *The Health of the Nation: A Strategy for Health in England*. London: HMSO.

Department of Health and Social Security (DHSS) (1976) *Prevention and Health: Everybody's Business*. London: HMSO.

Department of Social Security (DSS) (1998) *Building a Better Britain for Older People*. London: DSS.

Dill, A., Brown, P., Ciambrone, D. and Rakowski, W. (1995) The meaning and practice of self-care by older adults, *Research on Aging*, 17(1): 8–41.

Douglas, J. (1992) Black women's health matters: putting Black women on the research agenda, in H. Roberts (ed.) *Women's Health Matters*. London: Routledge.

Douglas, J. (1997) Developing health promotion strategies with Black and minority ethnic communities which address social inequalities, in M. Sidell, L. Jones, J. Katz and A. Peberdy (eds) *Debates and Dilemmas in Promoting Health: A Reader*. London: Macmillan.

Doyal, L. (1995) *What Makes Women Sick: Gender and the Political Economy of Health*. London: Macmillan.

Dychtwald, K. and Flower, J. (1989) *Age Wave: The Challenges and Opportunities of an Aging America*. New York: St Martin's Press.

Eadie, D., Stead, M. and Teer, P. (1996) The role of general practice in promoting physical activity as healthy lifestyle behaviour in older people, *Health Care in Later Life*, 1: 156–63.

Education and Ageing (1998) Special issue on the Work of the Beth Johnson Foundation 13(2).

Edwardson, M. (1993) Appropriateness: the neglected variable in self-care research. Paper presented to the World Congress of Gerontology, Budapest, Hungary, 4–9 July.

Elliott, J. (1980) *Action Research in Schools: Some Guidelines*, Classroom Action Research Network Bulletin no. 4. Norwich: University of East Anglia.

Ellis, S.W. (1998) *The Intergenerational Programme Mentoring Project: Final Research Report*. Stoke-on-Trent: Beth Johnson Foundation and Manchester Metropolitan University.

Ellis, S. and Noyes, K. (1990) *By the People: A History of Americans as Volunteers*. San Francisco, CA: Jossey-Bass.

Epp, J. (1986) Achieving health for all: a framework for health promotion, *Canadian Journal of Public Health*, 77(6): 393–430.

Estes, C.L., Gerard, L.E., Zones, J.S. and Swan, J.H. (1984) *Political Economy, Health and Aging*. Boston, MA: Little, Brown.

Evandrou, M. (1996) Health status of ethnic minorities. Paper presented to the British Society of Gerontology Annual Conference, Bristol, 19–22 September.

Evandrou, M. (ed.) (1997) *Baby Boomers: Ageing in the 21st Century*. London: Age Concern.

Evandrou, M. (1998) Great expectations: social policy and the new millennium elders, in M. Bernard and J. Phillips (eds) *The Social Policy of Old Age: Moving into the 21st Century*. London: Centre for Policy on Ageing.

Ewles, L. (1996) The impact of the NHS reforms on specialist health promotion in the NHS, in A. Scriven and J. Orme (eds) *Health Promotion: Professional Perspectives*. London: Macmillan.

Falkingham, J. (1997) Who are the baby boomers? A demographic profile, in M. Evandrou (ed.) *Baby Boomers: Ageing in the 21st Century*. London: Age Concern England.

Fawcett, S.B., White, G.W., Balcazar, F. *et al.* (1994) A contextual-behavioural model of empowerment: case studies involving people with disabilities, *American Journal of Community Psychology*, 22(4): 471–96.

Fawcett, S.B., Harris, K.J., Paine-Andrews, A.L. *et al.* (1995) *Reducing Risk for Chronic Disease: An Action Planning Guide for Community-Based Initiatives*. Lawrence, KS: University of Kansas Work Group on Health Promotion and Community Development.

Feek, W. (1988) *Working Effectively: A Guide to Evaluation Techniques*. London: Bedford Square Press.

Ferraro, K.F. (1987) Double jeopardy to health for black older adults?, *Journal of Gerontology*, 42(5): 538–53.

Fetterman, D.M., Kaftarian, S.J. and Wandersman, A. (eds) (1996) *Empowerment Evaluation: Knowledge and Tools for Self-assessment and Accountability*. London: Sage.

Fischer, L. and Schaffer, K.B. (1993) *Older Volunteers: A Guide to Research and Practice*. London: Sage.

Ford, G. and Taylor, R. (1985) The elderly as under-consulters: a critical reappraisal, *Journal of the Royal College of General Practitioners*, 35: 244–7.

Foster, P. (1995) *Women and the Health Care Industry*. Buckingham: Open University Press.

Foster, P. (1996) Women and health care, in C. Hallett (ed.) *Women and Social Policy: An Introduction*. Hemel Hempstead: Harvester Wheatsheaf.

Fox, J., Jones, D., Moser, I.R. and Goldblatt, P. (1985) Socio-economic differences in mortality, *Population Trends*, 40: 10–16.

Freidson, E. (1970) *Profession of Medicine*. New York: Dodd, Mead.

Freire, P. (1972) *The Pedagogy of the Oppressed*. London: Sheed and Ward.

Freire, P. (1973) *Education for Critical Consciousness*. New York: Seabury Press.

Freire, P. (1974) *Education and the Practice of Freedom*. London: Writers and Readers Publishing Cooperative.

Fries, J.F. (1980) Aging, natural death and the compression of morbidity, *New England Journal of Medicine*, 303(3): 130–5.

Fries, J.F. (1989) *Aging Well*. Reading, MA: Addison-Wesley.

Fries, J.F. (1990) Compression of morbidity: near or far?, *Milbank Memorial Fund Quarterly*, 67(2): 208–32.

Fries, J.F. (1993) Compression of morbidity 1993: life span, disability, and health care costs, *Facts and Research in Gerontology*, 7: 183–90.

Fries, J.F. (1996) Physical activity, the compression of morbidity, and the health of the elderly, *Journal of the Royal Society of Medicine*, 89(Feb.): 64–8.

Fries, J.F. and Crapo, L.M. (1981) *Vitality and Aging: Implications of the Rectangular Curve*. San Francisco, CA: W.H. Freeman.

Fries, J.F., Gukirpal, S., Morfeld, D., *et al.* (1994) Running and the development of disability with age, *Annals of Internal Medicine*, 121(7): 502–9.

Gartner, A. and Reissman, F. (1976) Health care in a technological age, in *Self-Help and Health: A Report*. New York: New Human Services Institute.

Generations – Journal of the American Society on Aging (1993) Special issue on Self-care and Older Adults, 17(3).

Gergen, K.J. (1985) The social constructionist movement in modern psychology, *American Psychologist*, 40(3): 266–75.

Ginn, J. and Arber, S. (1998) Gender and older age, in M. Bernard and J. Phillips (eds) *The Social Policy of Old Age: Moving into the 21st Century*. London: Centre for Policy on Ageing.

Ginn, G., Arber, S. and Cooper, H. (1997) *Researching Older People's Health Needs and Health Promotion Issues*. London: Health Education Authority.

Glendenning, F. (ed.) (1985) *New Initiatives in Self-Health Care for Older People*. Stoke-on-Trent: Beth Johnson Foundation in association with Department of Adult Education, Keele University and Health Education Council.

Glendenning, F. (ed.) (1986) *Working Together for Health: Older People and their Carers*. Stoke-on-Trent: Beth Johnson Foundation in association with Department of Adult Education, Keele University and Health Education Council.

Glendenning, F. and Percy, K. (eds) (1990) *Ageing, Education and Society: Readings in Educational Gerontology*. Stoke-on-Trent: Association for Educational Gerontology, Keele University.

Goldberg, D.P. (1972) *The Detection of Psychiatric Illness by Questionnaire*. London: Oxford University Press.

Grace, V.M. (1991) The marketing of empowerment and the construction of the health consumer: a critique of health promotion, *International Journal of Health Services*, 21: 329–43.

Granville, G. (1996) Promoting health in older people, in L. Wade and K. Waters (eds) *A Textbook of Gerontological Nursing: Perspectives on Practice*. London: Baillière Tindall.

Granville, G. (1998) The Foundation as a learning organisation: a model for responsible risk-taking and the empowerment of older people, *Education and Ageing*, 13(2): 163–76.

Greater London Association for Disabled People (GLAD) (1987) *Disability and Ethnic Minority Communities: A Study in Three London Boroughs*. London: GLAD.

Green, H. (1988) *Informal Carers*. OPCS series GHS no. 15, supplement A. London: HMSO.

Greengross, S. and Batty, M. (1989) *Elderly People and the Second European Programme to Combat Poverty: Final Review and Analysis*. Cologne: Transnational Team on Elderly People, ISG Sozialforschung und Gesellschaftspolitik.

Griffiths Report (1988) *Community Care: Agenda for Action*. London: HMSO.

Grimley Evans, J. (1993) Hypothesis: healthy active life expectancy (HALE) as an index of effectiveness of health and social services for elderly people, *Age and Ageing*, 22(4): 297–301.

Grimley Evans, J. (1998) A correct compassion: the medical response to an ageing society, the Harveian Oration of 1997, in R. Tallis (ed.) *Increasing Longevity: Medical, Social and Political Implications*. London: Royal College of Physicians.

Grimley Evans, J., Goldacre, M.J., Hodkinson, M., Lamb, S. and Savory, M. (1992) *Health: Abilities and Wellbeing in The Third Age*. Carnegie Enquiry into the Third Age, research paper no. 9. Dunfermline: Carnegie United Kingdom Trust.

Groombridge, J. (ed.) (1988) *Health Promotion and Older People*. London: Centre for Health and Retirement Education.

Grundy, E. (1996) Population Review 5: the population aged 60 and over, *Population Trends*, 84: 14–20.

Grundy, E. (1998) Ageing, ill health and disability, in R. Tallis (ed.) *Increasing Longevity: Medical, Social and Political Implications*. London: Royal College of Physicians.

Gubrium, J.F. and Sankar, A. (eds) (1994) *Qualitative Methods in Aging Research*. Thousand Oaks, CA: Sage.

Gutierrez, L. (1990) Working with women of color: an empowerment perspective, *Social Work*, 35: 149–54.

Hardey, M. (1998) *The Social Context of Health*. Buckingham: Open University Press.

Harding, S. (1986) *The Science Question in Feminism*. Milton Keynes: Open University Press.

Harding, S. (ed.) (1987) *Feminism and Methodology: Social Science Issues*. Milton Keynes: Open University Press.

Hart, E. and Bond, M. (1995) *Action Research for Health and Social Care: A Guide to Practice*. Buckingham: Open University Press.

Hatch, S. and Kickbusch, I. (eds) (1983) *Self-Help and Health in Europe: New Approaches in Health Care*. Copenhagen: World Health Organisation.

Health Education Authority (HEA)/Age Concern England (1988) *Age Well: Planning and Ideas Pack*. London: HEA.

Health Education Council (HEC) (1985) *Health Education and Promotion Among Older People: Planning Guidelines*. London: HEC.

HEC/Age Concern England (1985) *Age Well Ideas Pack*. London: HEC.

Hedley, R. (1985) *Measuring Success: A Guide to Evaluation for Voluntary and Community Groups*. London: ADVANCE.

Henwood, M. (1990) No sense of urgency, in E. McEwen (ed.) *Age: The Unrecognised Discrimination*. London: Age Concern England.

Herzlich, C. (1973) *Health and Illness: A Social Psychological Analysis*. London: Academic Press.

Herzog, A.R. and House, J.S. (1991) Productive activities and aging well, *Generations*, 1(3): 10–13.

Hickey, T. (1993) Self-care and health in old age. Symposium presented at the World Congress of Gerontology, Budapest, Hungary, 4–9 July.

Holstein, B.E. (1986) Health related behaviour and aging: conceptual issues, in K. Dean, T. Hickey and B.E. Holstein (eds) *Self-Care and Health in Old Age: Health Behaviour Implications for Policy and Practice*. London: Croom Helm.

Holter, I.M. and Schwartz-Barcott, D. (1993) Action research: what is it? How has it been used and how can it be used in nursing?, *Journal of Advanced Nursing*, 18: 298–304.

Hooyman, N.R. and Kiyak, H.A. (1988) *Social Gerontology*. Boston, MA: Allyn and Bacon.

Hopson, B. and Scally, M. (1981) *Lifeskills Teaching*. London: McGraw-Hill.

Huntington, J. (1985) Health Education Council: a programme of education for health in old age, in F. Glendenning (ed.) *New Initiatives in Self-Health Care for Older People*. Stoke-on-Trent: Beth Johnson Foundation in association with Department of Adult Education, Keele University and Health Education Council.

Iliffe, S., Patterson, L. and Gould, M.M. (1998) *Health Care for Older People*. London: BMJ Books.

Illsley, R. (1986) Preface, in K. Dean, T. Hickey and B.E. Holstein (eds) *Self-Care and Health in Old Age: Health Behaviour Implications for Policy and Practice*. London: Croom Helm.

Independent Sector (1988) *Giving and Volunteering in the United States: 1988 Edition*. Washington, DC: Independent Sector.

Ivers, V. (1985) New initiatives in North Staffordshire, in F. Glendenning (ed.) *New Initiatives in Self-Health Care for Older People*. Stoke-on-Trent: Beth Johnson Foundation in association with Department of Adult Education, Keele University and Health Education Council.

Ivers, V. and Meade, K. (1991) *Older Volunteers and Peer Health Counselling: A New Approach to Training and Development*. Stoke-on-Trent: Beth Johnson Foundation.

Jefferys, M. (1988) An Ageing Britain: what is its future?, in B. Gearing, M. Johnson and T. Heller (eds) *Mental Health Problems in Old Age: A Reader*. London: John Wiley.

Johnson, J. (1979a) *An Over 60s Day Centre: An Outline for its Setting Up and Development*. Stoke-on-Trent: Beth Johnson Foundation.

Johnson, J. (1979b) *A Mobile Day Centre for the Over 60s*. Stoke-on-Trent: Beth Johnson Foundation.

Johnson, M.L. (1998) Intergenerational equity: the politics and economics of an ageing population, in R. Tallis (ed.) *Increasing Longevity: Medical, Social and Political Implications*. London: Royal College of Physicians.

Jones, L. (1994) *The Social Context of Health and Health Work*. London: Macmillan.

Jones, L. (1997a) Health promotion and public policy, in L. Jones and M. Sidell (eds) *The Challenge of Promoting Health: Exploration and Action*. London: Macmillan.

Jones, L. (1997b) What is health?, in J. Katz and A. Peberdy (eds) *Promoting Health: Knowledge and Practice*. London: Macmillan in association with The Open University.

Jones, L. and Naidoo, J. (1997) Theories and models in health promotion, in J. Katz and A. Peberdy (eds) *Promoting Health: Knowledge and Practice*. London: Macmillan in association with The Open University.

Kalache, A., Warnes, T. and Hunter, D. (1988) *Promoting Health among Elderly People: A Health Promotion Challenge*. London: King Edward's Hospital Fund.

Katz, A.H. (1986) Self-care and self-help programmes for elders, in K. Dean, T. Hickey and B.E. Holstein (eds) *Self-Care and Health in Old Age: Health Behaviour Implications for Policy and Practice*. London: Croom Helm.

Katz, A.H. and Bender, E. (1976) *The Strength in Us: Self Help Groups in the Modern World*. New York: Franklin Watts.

Kelly, M. and Charlton, B. (1995) The modern and the post modern in health promotion, in R. Bunton, S. Nettleton and R. Burrows (eds) *The Sociology of Health Promotion: Critical Analyses of Consumption, Lifestyle and Risk*. London: Routledge.

Kennie, D. (1993) *Preventive Care for Elderly People*. Cambridge: Cambridge University Press.

Kickbusch, I. (1981) Involvement in Health: a concept of health education, *International Journal of Health Education*, 24 (Oct.–Dec.): 3.

Kickbusch, I. (1989) Self-care in health promotion, *Social Science and Medicine*, 29(2): 125–30.

Kickbusch, I. and Hatch, S. (1983) A re-orientation of health care?, in S. Hatch and I. Kickbusch (eds) *Self-Help and Health in Europe: New Approaches in Health Care*. Copenhagen: World Health Organisation.

Killoran, A., Howse, K. and Dalley, G. (1997) *Promoting the Health of Older People: A Compendium*. London: Health Education Authority.

Klein, R. (1989) *The Politics of the National Health Service*, 2nd edn. London: Longman.

Klein, R. (1995) *The New Politics of the National Health Service*, 3rd edn. London: Longman.

Knapp, M., Koutsogeorgopoulou, V. and Davis Smith, J. (1996) Volunteer participation in community care, *Policy and Politics*, 24(2): 171–92.

Knight, B. and Hayes, R. (1981) *Self-Help in the Inner City*. London: Voluntary Service Council.

Knight, B. and Hayes, R. (1982) *The Self Help Economy*. London: Voluntary Service Council.

Lalonde, M. (1974) *A New Perspective on the Health of Canadians*. Ottawa: Ministry of Supply and Services.

Lane, N.E., Bloch, D.A., Jones, H.H., *et al.* (1986) Long-distance running, bone density and osteoarthritis, *Journal of the American Medical Association*, 255: 1147–51.

Lane, N.E., Bloch, D.A., Wood, P.D. and Fries, J.F. (1987) Aging, long-distance running, and the development of musculoskeletal disability: a controlled study, *American Journal of Medicine*, 82: 772–80.

Lane, N.E., Bloch, D.A., Hubert, H.B., *et al.* (1990) Running, osteoarthritis, and bone density: initial 2-year longitudinal study, *American Journal of Medicine*, 88(5): 452–9.

Laslett, P. (1996) *A Fresh Map of Life*, 2nd edn. London: Macmillan.

Lathlean, J. (1994) Choosing an appropriate methodology, in J. Buckeldee and R. McMahon (eds) *The Research Experience in Nursing*. London: Chapman and Hall.

Leigh, J.P. and Fries, J.F. (1994) Education, gender, and the compression of morbidity, *International Journal of Aging and Human Development*, 39(3): 233–46.

Levin, L.S. (1982) *Yale Self-Care Education Project: Final Report*. New Haven, CT: Department of Epidemiology and Public Health, Yale University.

Levin, L.S. and Idler, E.L. (1981) *The Hidden Health Care System: Mediating Structures and Medicine*. Cambridge, MA: Ballinger.

Levin, L.S., Katz, A.H. and Holst, E. (1976) *Self-care: Lay Initiatives in Health*. New York: Prodist.

Levy, L.H. (1976) Self-help groups: types and psychological processes, *Journal of Applied Behavioural Science*, 12(summer): 312–13.

Lewin, K. (1946) Action research and minority problems, *Journal of Social Issues*, 2: 34–46.

Lewis, M. (1985) Older women and health: an overview, in S. Golub and R.J. Freedman (eds) *Health Needs of Women as They Age*. New York: Haworth Press.

Lincoln, Y.S. and Guba, E.G. (1985) *Naturalistic Inquiry*. London: Sage.

Lock, S. (1986) Self help groups: the fourth estate in medicine?, *British Medical Journal*, 293 (20–27 Dec): 1596–600.

Lorig, K. (1993) Self-management of chronic illness: a model for the future, *Generations*, XVII(3): 11–14.

Lynn, P. and Davis Smith, J. (1991) *The 1991 National Survey of Voluntary Activity in the UK*, Voluntary Action Research second series, paper no. 1. Berkhamsted: Volunteer Centre UK.

McClymont, M., Thomas, S. and Denham, M. (1991) *Health Visiting and Elderly People: A Health Promotion Challenge*. London: Longman.

MacDonald, T.H. (1998) *Rethinking Health Promotion: A Global Approach*. London: Routledge.

Macfadyen, D.M. (1985) New initiatives in self-health care for older people, in F. Glendenning (ed.) *New Initiatives in Self-Health Care for Older People*. Stoke-on-Trent: Beth Johnson Foundation in association with Department of Adult Education, Keele University and Health Education Council.

McKernan, J. (1989) Action research and curriculum development, *Peabody Journal of Education*, 64(2): 6–20.

McKernan, J. (1991) *Curriculum Action Research: A Handbook of Methods and Resources for the Reflective Practitioner*. London: Kogan Page.

McLeod, J. (1994) *Doing Counselling Research*. London: Sage

McNiff, J. (1988) *Action Research: Principles and Practice*. London: Macmillan Education.

McNiff, J. (1993) *Teaching as Learning: An Action Research Approach*. London: Routledge.

Manning, N. (1994) Health services: pressure, growth and conflict, in V. George and S. Miller (eds) *Social Policy Towards 2000: Squaring the Welfare Circle*. London: Routledge.

Manton, K.G. (1982) Changing concepts of mortality and morbidity in the elderly population, *Milbank Memorial Fund Quarterly/Health and Society*, 60: 183–244.

Manton, K.G. (1986) Past and future life expectancy increases at later ages: their implications for the linage of chronic morbidity, disability, and mortality, *The Gerontologist*, 41: 672–81.

Manton, K.G. and Stallard, E. (1994) Medical demography: interaction of disability dynamics and mortality, in L.G. Martin and S.H. Preston (eds) *Demography of Aging*. Washington, DC: National Academy Press.

Manton, K.G., Corder, L. and Stallard, E. (1997) Chronic disability trends in elderly United States populations: 1982–1994, *Proceedings of the National Academy of Science*, 94: 2593–8.

Marmot, M.G., Adelstein, A. and Bulusu, L. (1984) *Immigrant Mortality in England and Wales, 1970–78: Causes of Death by Country of Birth*, Studies on Medical and Population Subjects no. 47. London: HMSO.

Meade, K. (1986) *Challenging the Myths: A Review of Pensioners' Health Courses and Talks*. London: Age Well.

Meade, K. (1987) *Helping Yourself to Health – Health Courses for Older People: A 'How To' Guide*. London: Pensioners' Link and Health Education Council.

Meade, K. and Carter, T. (1990) Empowering older users: some starting points, in L. Winn (ed.) *Power to the People: The Key to Responsive Services in Health and Social Care*. London: King's Fund Centre.

Meadows, A. and Turkie, A. (1988) *How Are We Doing? An Introduction to Self-Evaluation for Voluntary Groups*. London: NCVO Inner Cities Unit.

Mettler, M. and Kemper, D.W. (1993) Self-care and older adults: making healthcare relevant, *Generations*, XVII(3): 7–10.

Midwinter, E. (1991) *The British Gas Report on Attitudes to Ageing 1991*. London: Burson-Marstellar.

Midwinter, E. (1994) *The Development of Social Welfare in Britain*. Buckingham: Open University Press.

Miles, A. (1988) *Women and Mental Illness*. Brighton: Wheatsheaf.

Minkler, M. (1985) Building supportive ties and sense of community among inner-city elderly: the Tenderloin Senior Outreach Project, *Health Education Quarterly*, 12(4): 303–14.

Minkler, M. (1992) Community organizing among the elderly poor in the United States: a case study, *International Journal of Health Services*, 22(2): 303–16.

Minkler, M. (1995) Critical perspectives on ageing: new challenges for gerontology. Paper presented to the British Society of Gerontology Annual Conference, Keele University, 15–17 September.

Minkler, M. (1996) Critical perspectives on ageing: new challenges for gerontology, *Ageing and Society*, 16(4): 467–87.

Mockenhaupt, R. (1993) Self-care for older adults: taking care and taking charge, *Generations*, XVII(3): 5–6.

MORI (1990) *Voluntary Activity: A Survey of Public Attitudes*. Berkhamsted: Volunteer Centre UK.

Munday, J. (1991) *New for Old: Volunteering in Retirement*. London: Retired Executive Action Clearing House.

Nathanson, C.A. (1977) Sex, illness and medical care: a review of data, theory and method, *Social Science and Medicine*, 11(1): 13–25.

National Institute on Aging (1984) *Self-Care and Self-Help Groups for the Elderly: A Directory*. Bethesda, MD: National Institute on Aging.

Nazroo, J. (1997) Health and health services, in T. Modood, R. Berthoud, *et al.* (eds) *Ethnic Minorities in Britain: Diversity and Disadvantage*. London: Policy Studies Institute.

Nettleton, S. and Bunton, R. (1995) Sociological critiques of health promotion, in R. Bunton, S. Nettleton and R. Burrows (eds) *The Sociology of Health Promotion and the New Public Health*. London: Routledge.

Newman, S., Ward, C.R., Smith, T.B., Wilson, J.O. and McCrea, J.M. (1997) *Intergenerational Programs: Past, Present and Future*. Washington, DC: Taylor & Francis.

NHS Centre for Reviews and Dissemination (1996) *Ethnicity and Health*. York: NHS Centre for Reviews and Dissemination.

Nixon, J. (1992) *Evaluating the Whole Curriculum*. Buckingham: Open University Press.

Nocerino, J., Pringle, J. and Sehnert, K. (1977) *Health Activation for Senior Citizens: A Course Guide*. Vienna, VA: Health Activation Network.

Nutbeam, D. (1998) Evaluating health promotion: progress, problems and solutions, *Health Promotion International*, 13(1): 27–43.

Nutbeam, D., Smith, C. and Catford, J. (1990) Evaluation in health education: a review of progress, possibilities and problems, *Journal of Epidemiology and Community Health*, 44: 83–9.

Office for National Statistics (ONS) (1996) *Population Trends 84*. London: HMSO.

Office of Health Economics (OHE) (1995) *Compendium of Health Statistics*. London: OHE.

Office of Population Censuses and Surveys (OPCS) (1993) *General Household Survey 1991*. London: OPCS.

OPCS (1995) *Health Survey for England 1993*. London: HMSO.

OPCS (1996) *Living in Britain: Report on the General Household Survey 1994*. London: HMSO.

OPCS (1997) *1994-Based National Population Projections*. London: HMSO.

Olshansky, S.J., Rudberg, M.A., Carnes, B.A., Cassel, C.K. and Brody, J.A. (1991) Trading off longer life for worsening health: the expansion of morbidity hypothesis, *Journal of Aging and Health*, 3(2): 194–216.

Parish, R. (1995) Health promotion: rhetoric and reality, in R. Bunton, S. Nettleton and R. Burrows (eds) *The Sociology of Health Promotion: Critical Analyses of Consumption, Lifestyle and Risk*. London: Routledge.

Peace, S. and Johnson, J. (1998) Living arrangements of older people, in M. Bernard and J. Phillips (eds) *The Social Policy of Old Age: Moving into the 21st Century*. London: Centre for Policy on Ageing.

Pederson, D. *et al.* (1988) Health policy in the Netherlands, *Health Promotion International*, 3.

Perry, N. (1977) The design and implementation of evaluation in the leisure experiments, in *Leisure and the Quality of Life: A Report on Four Local Experiments*, vol. 2. London: HMSO.

Petty, B.J. and Cusack, S.A. (1989) Assessing the impact of a community peer counselling program, *Educational Gerontology*, 15: 49–64.

Phillips, A. and Rakusen, J. (eds) (1989) *The New Our Bodies, Ourselves: A Health Book by and for Women*, British edition. Harmondsworth: Penguin.

Phillipson, C.R. (1984) Introduction – health education and older people: the role of self-care and self-help, in C. Savo (ed.) *Self-Care and Self-Help Programmes for Older Adults in the United States*, working papers on the health of older people no. 1. Stoke-on-Trent: Health Education Council in association with Department of Adult Education, Keele University.

Phillipson, C. and Strang, P. (1984) *Health Education and Older People: The Role of Paid Carers*. Stoke-on-Trent: Health Education Council in association with Department of Adult Education, Keele University.

Phillipson, C. and Strang, P. (1986) *Training and Education for an Ageing Society*. Stoke-on-Trent: Health Education Council in association with Department of Adult Education, Keele University.

Phillipson, C., Bernard, M., Phillips, J. and Ogg, J. (1998) *The Family and Community Life of Older People: Social Networks and Social Support in Three Urban Areas*, Research Results no. 9 (June). Swindon: ESRC Population and Household Change Research Programme.

Piachaud, D. (1987) Problems in the definition and measurement of poverty, *Journal of Social Policy*, 16(2): 147–64.

Pietroni, P.C. (1995) The greening of medicine, in B. Davey, A. Gray and C. Seale (eds) *Health and Disease: A Reader*, 2nd edn. Buckingham: Open University Press.

Pill, R. and Stott, N.C.H. (1982) Concept of illness causation and responsibility: some preliminary data from a sample of working-class mothers, *Social Science and Medicine*, 16: 43–52.

Pill, R. and Stott, N.C.H. (1985) Preventive procedures and practices among working-class women: new data and fresh insights, *Social Science and Medicine*, 21: 975–83.

Popay, J. *et al.* (1993) The impact of industrialisation on world health, in A. Beattie, M. Gott, L.J. Jones and M. Sidell (eds) *Health and Wellbeing: A Reader*. London: Macmillan.

Posner, T. (1989) The development of self help organisations: dilemmas and ambiguities, in S. Humble and J. Unell (eds) *Self Help in Health and Social Welfare: England and West Germany*. London: Routledge.

Public Health Alliance (PHA) (1994) *Poverty and Health*. Birmingham: PHA.

Qureshi, H. and Walker, A. (1989) *The Caring Relationship: Elderly People and their Families*. London: Macmillan.

Rakowski, W. and Hickey, T. (1980) Later life health behaviour, *Research on Aging*, 2(3): 283–308.

Raleigh, V., Kiri, V. and Balarajan, R. (1996) Variations in mortality from diabetes mellitus, hypertension and renal disease in England and Wales by country of birth, *Health Trends*, 28: 122–7.

Rappaport, J. (1981) In praise of paradox: a social policy of empowerment over prevention, *American Journal of Community Psychology*, 9: 1–25.

Rappaport, J. (1984) Studies in empowerment: introduction to the issue, *Prevention in Human Services*, 3: 1–7.

Rappaport, J. (1987) Terms of empowerment/exemplars of prevention: toward a theory for community psychology, *American Journal of Community Psychology*, 15(2): 121–48.

Rappaport, J., Swift, C. and Hess, R. (eds) (1984) *Studies in Empowerment: Steps towards Understanding and Action*. New York: Haworth.

Reason, P. (ed.) (1988) *Human Inquiry in Action: Developments in New Paradigm Research*. London: Sage.

Reason, P. (1994) *Participation in Human Inquiry*. London: Sage.

Reason, P. and Rowan, J. (eds) (1981) *Human Inquiry: A Source Book of New Paradigm Research*. Chichester: Wiley.

Reinharz, S. (1992) *Feminist Methods in Social Research*. Oxford: Oxford University Press.

Richardson, A. and Goodman, M. (1983) *Self-Help and Health: Mutual Aid for Modern Problems*. London: Martin Robertson.

Rissel, C. (1994) Empowerment: the holy grail of health promotion?, *Health Promotion International*, 9(1): 39–47.

Robbins, D. (1987a) *Monitoring and Evaluation: Report of a Seminar Held on 2–3 October 1986*. Bath: Centre for the Analysis of Social Policy, University of Bath.

Robbins, D. (1987b) Signs of poverty. Unpublished paper presented to the Conference on the European Programme Against Poverty: Action in the UK, UK Forum on Poverty in the EEC, Wolverhampton, 16–18 December.

Roberts, H. (1985) *The Patient Patients*. London: Pandora Press.

Robinson, R. and Judge, K. (1987) *Public Expenditure and the NHS: Trends and Prospects*. London: King's Fund Institute.

Rogers, A., Rogers, R.G. and Belanger, A. (1990) Longer life but worse health? Measurement and dynamics, *The Gerontologist*, 30(5): 640–9.

Room, G. (1990) *Final Report of the Programme Evaluation Team*. Bath: Centre for the Analysis of Social Policy and Cologne, ISG Sozialforschung und Gesellschaftspolitik.

Royal Association for Disability and Rehabilitation (RADAR) (1984) *Disability and Minority Ethnic Groups: A Fact Sheet of Issues and Initiatives*. London: RADAR.

Royal College of General Practitioners (RCGP) with OPCS and DHSS (1986) *Morbidity Statistics from General Practice*, Third National Study 1981/2. London: HMSO.

Rudat, K. (1994) *Health and Lifestyles: Black and Minority Ethnic Groups in England*. London: Health Education Authority.

Sanders, G.S. (1982) Social comparison and perceptions of health and illness, in G.S. Sanders and J. Suls (eds) *Social Psychology of Health and Illness*. Hillsdale, NJ: Lawrence Erlbaum.

Sapsford, R. and Abbott, P. (1992) *Research Methods for Nurses and the Caring Professions*. Buckingham: Open University Press.

Savo, C. (1983) Self care and empowerment: a case study, *Social Policy*, 14(1): 19–22.

Savo, C. (1984) *Self-Care and Self-Help Programmes for Older Adults in the United States*, working papers on the health of older people no. 1. Stoke-on-Trent: Health Education Council in association with Department of Adult Education, Keele University.

Savo, C. (1985) New developments in self-health care in America, in F. Glendenning (ed.) *New Initiatives in Self-Health Care for Older People*. Stoke-on-Trent: Beth Johnson

Foundation in association with Department of Adult Education, Keele University and Health Education Council.

Scambler, A., Scambler, G. and Craig, D. (1981) Kinship and friendship networks and women's demand for primary care, *Journal of the Royal College of General Practitioners*, 26: 746–50.

Schneider, E.L. and Brody, J.A. (1983) Aging, natural death and the compression of morbidity: another view, *New England Journal of Medicine*, 309: 854.

Scrutton, S. (1992) *Ageing, Healthy and in Control: An Alternative Approach to Maintaining the Health of Older People*. London: Chapman and Hall.

Sehnert, K.W. and Eisenberg, H. (1975) *How To Be Your Own Doctor (Sometimes)*. New York: Grosset and Dunlap.

Shapiro, J. (ed.) (1989) *Ourselves, Growing Older: Women Ageing with Knowledge and Power*, British edition. London: Fontana/Collins.

Sharma, U. (1995) Using alternative therapies: marginal medicine and central concerns, in B. Davey, A. Gray and C. Seale (eds) *Health and Disease: A Reader*, 2nd edn. Buckingham: Open University Press.

Sidell, M. (1991) *Gender Differences in the Health of Older People*, research report. Milton Keynes: Department of Health and Social Welfare, The Open University.

Sidell, M. (1992) The relationship of elderly women to their doctors, in J. George and S. Ebrahim (eds) *Health Care for Older Women*. Oxford: Oxford University Press.

Sidell, M. (1993) Health issues and the older woman, in M. Bernard and K. Meade (eds) *Women Come of Age: Perspectives on the Lives of Older Women*. London: Edward Arnold.

Sidell, M. (1995) *Health in Old Age: Myth, Mystery and Management*. Buckingham: Open University Press.

Sidell, M. (1997) Partnerships and collaborations: the promise of participation, in L. Jones and M. Sidell (eds) *The Challenge of Promoting Health: Exploration and Action*. London: Macmillan in association with The Open University.

Silten, R.M. and Levin, L.S. (1979) Self-care education, in P.M. Lazes (ed.) *Handbook of Health Education*, Germantown, MD: Aspen Systems Corporation.

Silveira, E. and Ebrahim, S. (1995) Mental health and health status of elderly Bengalis and Somalis in London, *Age and Ageing*, 24(6): 474–80.

Social Science and Medicine (1989) Special issue on 'self-care', 29(2).

Sparrow, S. and Robinson, J. (1994) Action research: an appropriate design for research in nursing?, *Educational Action Research*, 2(3): 347–55.

Sports Council (1982) *Sport in the Community: The Next Ten Years*. London: Sports Council.

Stainton-Rogers, W. (1991) *Explaining Health and Illness: An Exploration of Diversity*. Hemel Hempstead: Harvester.

Stanley, L. (ed.) (1990) *Feminist Praxis*. London: Routledge.

Staples, L.H. (1990) Powerful ideas about empowerment, *Administration in Social Work*, 14(2): 29–42.

Stead, M., Wimbush, E., Eadie, D. and Teer, P. (1997) A qualitative study of older people's perceptions of ageing and exercise: the implications for health promotion, *Health Education Journal*, 56(1): 3–16.

Stevenson, C. and Cooper, N. (1996) A reconciling framework, in N. Cooper, C. Stevenson and G. Hale (eds) *Integrating Perspectives on Health*. Buckingham: Open University Press.

Stevenson, O. and Parsloe, P. (1993) *Community Care and Empowerment*. York: Joseph Rowntree Foundation.

Strauss, A. and Corbin, J. (1998) *Basics of Qualitative Research: Techniques and Procedures for Developing Grounded Theory*, 2nd edn. Thousand Oaks, CA: Sage.

Susman, G.I. and Evered, R.D. (1978) An assessment of the scientific merits of action research, *Administrative Science Quarterly*, 23: 582–603.

Tallis, R. (1998) Editor's introduction, in R. Tallis (ed.) *Increasing Longevity: Medical, Social and Political Implications*. London: Royal College of Physicians.

Tannahill, A. (1985) What is health promotion?, *Health Education Journal*, 44: 167–8.

Taylor, S. and Field, D. (1997) *Sociology of Health and Health Care: An Introduction for Nurses*, 2nd edn. Oxford: Blackwell Scientific.

Thursz, D., Nusberg, C. and Prather, J. (eds) (1995) *Empowering Older People: An International Approach*. London: Cassell.

Tinker, A. (1992) *Elderly People in Modern Society*, 3rd edn. London: Longman.

Titley, J. (1997) *Healthcare Rights for Older People: The Ageism Issue*. London: Age Concern England.

Tones, B.K. (1976) *Effectiveness and Efficiency in Health Education*. Edinburgh: Scottish Health Education Group.

Tones, B.K. (1979) Past achievement and future success, in I. Sutherland (ed.) *Health Education: Perspectives and Choices*. London: George Allen & Unwin.

Tones, B.K. (1981) Health education: prevention or subversion?, *Royal Society of Health Journal*, 101: 114–17.

Tones, B.K. (1983) Education and health promotion: new directions, *Journal of the Institute of Health Education*, 21: 121–3.

Tones, B.K. (1996) The anatomy and ideology of health promotion: empowerment in context, in A. Scriven and J. Orme (eds) *Health Promotion: Professional Perspectives*. London: Macmillan.

Tones, B.K. and Tilford, S. (1994) *Health Education: Effectiveness, Efficiency and Equity*, 2nd edn. London: Chapman and Hall.

Tout, K. (ed.) (1993) *Elderly Care: A World Perspective*. London: Chapman and Hall.

Townsend, P. (1987) Deprivation, *Journal of Social Policy*, 16(2): 125–46.

Townsend, P. and Davidson, N. (eds) (1986) *Inequalities in Health: The Black Report*. Harmondsworth: Penguin.

Townsend, P., Phillimore, P. and Beattie, A. (1988) *Health and Deprivation: Inequality and the North*. London: Croom Helm.

Tozer, R. and Thornton, P. (1995) *A Meeting of Minds: older people as research advisers*, Social Policy Reports no. 3. York: Social Policy Research Unit, York University.

Tracy, G.S. and Gussow, Z. (1976) Self-help groups: a grass-roots response to a need for services, *Journal of Applied Behavioural Science*, 12 (summer): 381–96.

Turner, L. and Willis, E. (1987) *Measuring Up: Guidelines in the Self-Evaluation of Volunteer Projects*. Berkhamsted: Volunteer Centre/National Federation of Community Organizations.

Twelvetrees, A. (1982) *Community Work*. London: Macmillan and British Association of Social Workers.

Twigg, J. (1998) Informal care of older people, in M. Bernard and J. Phillips (eds) *The Social Policy of Old Age: Moving into the 21st Century*. London: Centre for Policy on Ageing.

Ussher, J. (1989) *The Psychology of the Female Body*. London: Routledge.

Verbrugge, L.M. (1984) Longer life but worsening health? Trends in health and mortality of middle-aged and older persons, *Milbank Memorial Fund Quarterly/Health and Society*, 62(3): 475–519.

Verbrugge, L.M. (1989) Gender, aging and health, in K.S. Markides (ed.) *Aging and Health: Perspectives on Gender, Race, Ethnicity and Class*. Newbury Park, CA: Sage.

Vickery, D.M. and Levinson, A. (1993) The limits of self-care, *Generations*, XVII(3): 53–6.

Victor, C. (1991) *Health and Health Care in Later Life*. Buckingham: Open University Press.

Vincent, J. (1986) *Constraints on the Stability and Longevity of Self Help Groups in the Field of Health Care*. Loughborough: Centre for Research in Social Policy.

Walker, A. (1998) Speaking for themselves: the new politics of old age in Europe, *Education and Ageing*, 13(1): 13–36.

Walker, A. and Warren, L. (1996) *Changing Services for Older People: The Neighbourhood Support Units Innovation*. Buckingham: Open University Press.

Warnes, A.M. (1998) Population ageing over the next few decades, in R. Tallis (ed.) *Increasing Longevity: Medical, Social and Political Implications*. London: Royal College of Physicians.

Webb, C. (1990) Partners in research, *Nursing Times*, 86(32): 40–4.

Webb, R. (1990) The origins and aspirations of practitioner research, in R. Webb (ed.) *Practitioner Research in the Primary School*. Basingstoke: Falmer Press.

Webster, C. (1991) The elderly and the early National Health Service, in M. Pelling and R.M. Smith (eds) *Life, Death and the Elderly: Historical Perspectives*. London: Routledge.

Wells, N. and Freer, C. (eds) (1988) *The Ageing Population: Burden or Challenge?* London: Macmillan.

Wenger, G.C. (1988) *Old People's Health and Experience of the Caring Services: Accounts from Rural Communities in North Wales*. Liverpool: Liverpool University Press.

Whitaker, D.S. and Archer, J.L. (1989) *Research by Social Workers: Capitalising on Experience*. London: CCETSW (Central Council for the Education and Training of Social Workers).

Whitehead, M. (1987) *The Health Divide*. Harmondsworth: Penguin.

Williams, G. (1989) Hope for the humblest? The role of self-help in chronic illness: the case of ankylosing spondylitis, *Sociology of Health and Illness*, 11: 135–59.

Williams, R.G.A. (1981) Logical analysis as qualitative method I and II, *Sociology of Health and Illness*, 3(2): 140–87.

Williams, R.G.A. (1983) Concepts of health: an analysis of lay logic, *Sociology*, 17: 185–205.

Williams, R.G.A. (1990) *The Protestant Legacy: Attitudes to Death and Illness among Older Aberdonians*. Oxford: Oxford University Press.

World Health Organization (WHO) (1948) Preamble of the Constitution of the World Health Organization. Geneva: WHO.

World Health Organization (1977) *Health for All by the Year 2000*. Geneva: WHO.

World Health Organization (1978) *Primary Health Care*, Report of the International Conference on Primary Health Care, Alma Ata, USSR, 6–12 September 1978. Geneva: WHO.

World Health Organization (1984) *Report of the Working Group on Concepts and Principles of Health Promotion*. Copenhagen: WHO.

World Health Organization (1985) *Health For All in Europe by the Year 2000, Regional Targets*. Copenhagen: WHO.

Zimmerman, M. (1995) Psychological Empowerment: Issues and Illustrations, *American Journal of Community Psychology*, 23: 581–99.

Index

Note: page numbers in *italic* refer to illustrations

HEALTH IN OLD AGE
MYTH, MYSTERY AND MANAGEMENT

Moyra Sidell

- Why do many older people rate their health as good when 'objective' evidence suggests that old age is a time of inevitable decline and disease?
- How do different perspectives on health inform our understanding of health in old age?
- What are the policy implications for ensuring a healthy future for old age?

This book addresses important questions which existing literature on health and old age has largely ignored. By juxtaposing detailed case histories and first person accounts from older people with 'official statistics' on the health of 'the elderly' it explores the myths and tries to unpick the mysteries which surround the subject of health in later life. It goes on to explore the implications of these myths and mysteries for the way individual older people manage their health. It looks at the resources and social support available to them as well as the implications for public policy provision. The book ends by exploring the problems and possibilities of ensuring a healthy future for old age. It will be essential reading for reflective practitioners and for anyone concerned with new developments in the fields of ageing, social policy and health.

Contents
Introduction – Part 1: The health context – The mirage of health – Lay logic – Patterns of health and illness among older people – Part 2: Experiencing health – Understanding chronic illness and disability – Maintaining health with physical illness and functional disability – Maintaining health with mental malaise – Part 3: Resources for health – Health care and the management of health – Personal resources and social support – A healthy future for old age – Bibliography – Index.

200pp   0 335 19136 3 (Paperback)   0 335 19336 6 (Hardback)

OLDER PEOPLE AND COMMUNITY CARE
CRITICAL THEORY AND PRACTICE

Beverley Hughes

Older People and Community Care sets social and health care practice with older people firmly in the context of the new community care arrangements and the consequent organizational trends towards a market culture. However, it also questions the relative lack of attention given by professionals to issues of structural inequality in old age, compared for example to race and gender. Thus, the book tackles a double agenda.

• How can community care practice be suffused with anti-ageist values and principles?

Addressing this question the book sets out the foundation knowledge and values which must underpin the development of anti-discriminatory community care practice and examines the implications for practitioners in terms of the essential skills and inherent dilemmas which arise.

Older People and Community Care is essential reading for all those working with and managing services to older people, and who aspire to make empowerment for older people a reality.

Contents
Introduction: understanding the NHS and Community Care Act – Part 1: Knowledge and values: Theories of ageing – The social condition of older people – Ageism and anti-ageist practice – Part 2: Skills – Communicating with older people: the professional encounter – Assessment – Implementing and managing care – Direct work with users and carers – Protection – Conclusion: challenges and priorities – References – Index.

176pp   0 335 19156 8 (Paperback)   0 335 19157 6 (Hardback)